THE TEN-POINT WAY TO HEALTH

THE TEN-POINT WAY TO HEALTH

SURYA NAMASKARS

SHRINIWASRAO PANT PRATINIDHI

GYAN

Published by

Gyan Publishing House
5, Ansari Road
Daryaganj, New Delhi-110002
Phone: 011-47034999, 9811692060
E-mail: books@gyanbooks.com

Distribution Network
gyanbooks.com
India, USA, Canada, UK, Australia

ISBN: 978-93-7225-038-1 (PB)

First Published, 1945

2nd Impression 2025

Printed at: Gyan Press, Delhi.

THE TEN-POINT WAY TO HEALTH
Author: SHRINIWASRAO PANT PRATINIDHI

THE TEN-POINT WAY TO HEALTH

THE TEN-POINT WAY TO HEALTH

SURYA NAMASKARS

Shrimant Balasahib Pandit Pratinidhi, B.A.
RAJAH OF AUNDH

20 ILLUSTRATIONS

CONTENTS

INTRODUCTION

I

A LITTLE over a year ago, in my capacity as journalist, I had the privilege of talking with one of the most vital human beings I have ever met —and I have interviewed hundreds of the world's outstanding men and women.

He is the Rajah of Aundh, ruling prince of one of the states in the Bombay Presidency, a wise legislator and humanitarian, who is rebuilding his domain into a modern progressive state from which old age, pain, disease, worry, and economic ills are being gradually eliminated.

I had discovered beforehand that the rajah was over seventy, and knowing that Indians age early, I was prepared for even more of the sagging muscles and profound wrinkles which mark the vast majority of 'old people' everywhere.

Imagine my astonishment, therefore, when the rajah's secretary presented me to him in the drawing-room of a suite at the Savoy Hotel, to see a man with the agile, supple movements of youth, eyes shining like a boy's, strong, brilliantly white teeth, firm muscles, radiant smile, and a mind that worked like summer lightning.

He looked a young middle-age. Later he was to tell me that he had known no illness, not even a cold, for twenty-eight years.

'You seem surprised not to find me the usual doddering old creature!' he said, and his secretary joined in our laugh. It was impossible to resist the good humour of this young man of seventy-one.

2

The rajah then told me a story of healing and the renewing of the life force which sounded like the discovery of the long-sought Fountain of Youth.

But the secret was nothing so miraculous; it lay in a series of exercises called 'Surya Namaskars,' literally translated 'Sun Prayers.'

They were simplicity itself, he explained, taking only five or six minutes to complete a round of twenty-five cycles and requiring no sort of equipment whatever.

Breathing was a fundamental part of Surya Namaskars, three controlled breaths being taken for each cycle of ten positions.

Any one could try them, of any age, men or women alike. They cost nothing, all that was necessary being a flat floor space about two feet by seven feet.

The rajah had brought with him a film taken

in his palace and in his state schools showing himself, his ranee, children, and subjects going through the exercises, and I was shown 'stills' from it.

The ranee, a charming woman of thirty-six who has had eight children, looked like a girl of sixteen. Her body was slender, supple, and delicately rounded. I was told she is extremely strong and suffers practically no pain at childbirth.

'The effect of Surya Namaskars on women is even more astonishing than on men,' said the rajah. 'Our women age very rapidly, but now they can keep the vitality and beauty of their youth to an advanced age.'

Another woman actor in the film was the sixty-year-old mother of ten children, who had suffered all her life from rheumatism and superfluous fat. She began the Namaskars in 1925, and had completely got rid of her rheumatism and was now 'as young-looking as her daughters.'

3

I was deeply impressed with the rajah's story, but, being a sceptical newspaperwoman, not entirely convinced. So when I returned to the office of my paper, the *News Chronicle*, to write the interview for the next day's issue, I did not sign it, for to sign it would have implied more credence than I felt.

A year earlier, and I should soon have forgotten both rajah and story in the whirl of Fleet Street, where one event tops another in the course of an hour or even less.

But, as it happened, I had had a twelvemonth of unusual stresses and strains, and was for the first time aware of a possible drain on the abundant capital of energy with which Nature had supplied me.

Also, I was on the eve of my holiday. The image of the ageless man went with me to the Dorset coast, and there I found myself one morning trying Surya Namaskars in the spirit in which the rajah had described them to me.

From the very first I noted a reflow of energy back into my being. Pursuing them with too much vigour, I strained several muscles, so that I limped for days. But, in spite of this, I persisted, and in six weeks' time I understood the significance of many sayings of the rajah which had been obscure to me.

Meanwhile, letters had been pouring into the *News Chronicle* office, requiring further information in regard to the 'fountain of youth' and the 'ten-point way to health'—the exercises described in my interview with the rajah, and as a result I was asked by the editor to write a series giving full particulars of Surya Namaskars.

This brought me in touch with a twenty-three-year-old son of the rajah studying law in London for the purpose of helping his father in his state work.

Shrimant Appasahib was a magnificent physical specimen, but there was about him a more impressive quality than perfect bodily fitness. He had, in the midst of nerve-ridden London, an Olympian calmness and poise.

He had practised Surya Namaskars since he was a small boy, and to them he attributed the fact that he had never had an illness and never known such a thing as fear. I watched him pose for the photographs at the end of this book, and when he had finished the dozen or so Namaskars necessary he was dripping and radiant as if he had risen out of some eternal spring.

The great advantage of these exercises, he told me, is that they do not strain any part of the body, or over-develop some muscles at the expense of others, but they search out every cell and sinew, rousing them, and tuning them into harmony. They 'make the body sing.'

In this way Shrimant Appasahib used them as a tonic immediately after a hard day's sport, such as ski-ing, to prevent soreness and fatigue.

They had also kept his nerves in good condition for his law examinations, he told me, removing all trace of uneasiness and clearing his brain.

4

The *News Chronicle* series illustrated with photographs of Shrimant Appasahib appeared in August 1936, and now, over a year later, I still receive letters regularly from people all over the country and abroad who have been carrying out the exercises and deriving benefit from them. They have told me of remarkable cures, of the restoration of faith and hope, and of the intensification of emotional experience which made each waking to a new day a delight.

These letters come from a representative section of the readers of a great national newspaper—doctors, school teachers, bankers and bank clerks, poets, saxophonists, newspaper vendors, charwomen, typists, retired civil servants, writers, engineers, actors, and dozens of other types.

One letter touched me more than most, and I reproduce it here, omitting only the name and address:

DEAR SIR,

Having been a reader of your paper for a number of years I should like to thank Louise Morgan through your paper for the Surya Namaskars.

First of all, I have been a miner and have worked

at —— Collieries since the age of 18 and am now 52, nearly all that time having been spent crutting, that is driving tunnels from one seam of coal to another using compressed air engine which you hold against the body for boring holes which are afterwards charged with Powder and then fired. You clean up and carry on till Coal is reached. Sometimes the rock is so hard it will take over an hour to bore it one yard. Just think of the dust which is not allowed to settle owing to the Caffling about of the exhaust and with all the latest devices. A man must breathe a big percentage of dust. For every shot thats fired the concussion picks up dust fifty yards away. No wonder three of my mates have died before the age of forty-three. About my own health, on Feb 22nd 1936 I had to give up work owing to Silicosis having been X-rayed and found well-established in both lungs. I am receiving Compensation weekly for same.

When visiting my Panel Doctor which is one and a half miles away there is a steep bank for about sixty yards. Every time I have gone that way I have had to stop halfway for a few seconds to get my breath, now I can walk pretty sharp all the way to the Doctors without any effect.

I happened to read Louise Morgan's first article of exercises but didn't think any thing of it till the next morning as I lay in bed too tired to get up thinking and wishing I could do 100 yards in twenty seconds, then I thought about lungs that were idle, could I get them to work. So I slipped out of bed and stood in position, now draw in count seven, I did, when up to three I was done but I kept on puffing out till I counted four and after following it up every morning as soon as I get out of bed I feel that much better I can count nine now and instead of two hours in the green fields which used to knock me up I can do six without being extra tired. The doctor tells me I shall be able to work again in a few years time.

Will fellow sufferers just think of it, nerves better, mental worry gone, just try the breathing exercises.

If you would like to take copy of Certificate, will forward it on to you.

Shake hands with Louise Morgan for me as I feel a new man.

Yours faithfully,

—

The testimony of these unsolicited letters, covering a period of over a year, added to my own personal experiment, has convinced me that Surya Namaskars have a healing, strengthening, and revitalizing effect on the entire being—on mind and spirit as well as body.

They help women equally with men because their aim is to free to the fullest extent the individual personality.

Some explanation of their power may be found in the fact that they are the concentration of hundreds of generations of human experience. The rajah emphasizes their ancient and traditional origin; he himself has but improved and adapted them.

They include the full cycle of human activity since the casting-out from the Garden of Eden;

the thrusting down of the treader of grapes and the woman in childbirth, the proud stretch of the warrior and the coquette, the swing of reaper and weaver, the tautness of runner and mother protecting her young, the bend of the weeder, the washer, and the human being at prayer.

In our mechanized times, these natural physical movements have been lost or distorted, and it restores something of the primitive vigour and oneness of being to revive them.

We westerners are a young people. The East goes back a very long way!

5

Sound is always associated with movement in eastern exercises. The recitation of the *mantras*, which are certain syllables so ancient that they have lost their meaning, invariably accompanies the ritual of health or religion.

But the rajah desires most sincerely to have it known that the furthest thing from his mind is any kind of proselytizing purpose.

The *mantras* are essentially non-religious, and owe none of their virtues to a religious source. Instead of the *mantras* themselves (*hram*, *hrim*, *hrum*, *hraim*, *hraum*, *hrah*), the separate vowels or consonants of which they are compounded may be spoken with exactly as good effect.

6

The present edition of *Surya Namaskars* is the fourth. The other three were published in India in 1928, 1929, and 1931, and each edition was out of print a few months after publication.

So sure was the faith of the rajah in Surya Namaskars to improve the physical, mental, and spiritual condition of mankind, that he published the book out of his private purse. Whatever moneys accrued from the sale of the book were devoted to welfare work among the youth of his state. The rajah's share in the present edition will be devoted to the same object in this country.

I wish to thank Mr Gerald Barry, editor of the *News Chronicle*, for allowing me to reprint the photographs of Shrimant Appasahib taken from the series of articles published in August 1936.

I should like also to express my appreciation of the kind help given me by Mr S. N. Dutt of India House in adapting the Indian terminology.

L. M.

1938.

THE TEN-POINT WAY TO HEALTH

CHAPTER I

THE HABIT OF HEALTH

Most people think that if they did more business, they would enjoy life better, but they do not appreciate the fact that if they enjoyed life better they would do more business.

Unless they are healthy they can never enjoy life.

Man's first duty, therefore, is to acquire superb health. Your success financially, socially, and personally depends fundamentally on your health.

The annual loss to industry and commerce, not to mention the privation entailed on individual families, brought about by illness and physical inefficiency on the part of workers is beyond computation.

The philosopher Emerson says: 'The first wealth is health. Sickness is poor-spirited and cannot serve any one; it must husband its resources to live. But health or fullness answers its own ends, and has to spare, runs over and inundates the neighbourhoods and creeks of other men's necessities.'

The time has now come for some strenuous

effort to be made in all seriousness to overcome the national degeneracy, and economic inefficiency all over the world, due to bad health.

Until now, a number of different ways and methods have been tried with but small success. In spite of the advance of medical science, old diseases are on the increase and new ones are coming into existence.

All this is due to the inexcusable and profoundly culpable neglect of the wise maxim, 'Prevention is better than cure.' Our chief energy should now be directed towards adopting measures to prevent rather than to cure disease. This is the only way to break the vicious chain of heredity, which passes on the ill health of the father and mother to the children. Create a race of healthy fathers and mothers, and you will have healthy children. Let us forget our unhappy generation and build for the future.

Some scientific and systematic form of bodily exercise, adopted to develop young bodies to their perfection, should therefore at once be enforced upon the younger generation in general, and upon young people in particular in schools, colleges, and universities.

There are no short cuts or specifics for health. It must be acquired and maintained throughout life by the observance of a rigid regimen. From our long observation and personal experience we are convinced that some sort of persistent effort is required on the part of the individual for him or her to grow strong and healthy, and to remain so.

The great thing is to create the habit of health in youth.

Physical exercise has always been, and still is, necessary to the human being for health. It is as necessary to life as water, food, air, and sunshine. In the present terrible struggle for existence it is indispensable to every modern individual, so that he may be able to support himself and his family and be a help rather than a hindrance to his community and to the world.

Almost all children, until they are about eight years old, amuse themselves by running about and romping and by playing a variety of outdoor and indoor games. They are usually so active that they keep their muscular system in fairly good tone and their various functions fairly normal. When, however, children are confined in schoolrooms for hours on end and the chubbiness of infancy begins to disappear to make way for further bodily development, they must be made to take some methodical exercise every day without fail.

Until a boy or girl knows how absolutely

CHAPTER II

THE MEANING OF SURYA NAMASKARS

Is there a universal kind of exercise, right for all ages, for children and women as well as for men, costing nothing, and capable of being performed in a short time, without accessories, at any moment, anywhere?

There is, and it is called Surya Namaskars. Our Indian readers would know at once what we mean. But to western readers we must explain.

'Surya Namaskars' are literally translated 'sun obeisances' or 'sun prayers.' They go back thousands of years. Then, as now, man looked to the sun for light, warmth, health, hygiene, and food. The sun purified things that had festered or moulded or accumulated disease-germs in the dark. The sun caused the growth and ripening of grain, fruit, and other foods by which man sustained life. To early man, the sun was the life-giver, and the thinkers and sages of India thousands of years ago showed their gratitude by making obeisances (or doing exercises) at the rising and the setting of the sun.

They bowed to the sun as you would to-day to one who had bestowed so many priceless gifts on humanity.

'Sun worship' is anathema to many westerners because they do not rightly understand it. But the great German philosopher and scientist, Ernst Haeckel, knew the reality which lies behind the sun-symbol. He wrote:

> The sun is the deity of light and warmth, on whose influence all organic life insensibly and directly depends. Sun-worship (solarism or heliotheism) seems to the modern scientist to be the best of all forms of theism, and the one which may be most easily reconciled with modern monism. For modern astrophysics and geogeny have taught us that the earth is a fragment detached from the sun, and that it will eventually return to the bosom of its parent. . . . Indeed the whole of our bodily and mental life depends, in the last resort, like all other organic life, on the light and heat of the sun. . . . As a matter of fact the sun-worshippers attained thousands of years ago a higher intellectual and moral standard than most of the other theists. When I was in Bombay in 1881 I watched with the greatest sympathy the elevating rites of the pious Parsees, who standing on the seashore, or kneeling on their prayer-rugs, offered their devotion to the sun at its rise and setting.

Let us emphasize here, for those who would be inclined to object to Surya Namaskars on the ground that they are a religious rite, *that they have the appearance only of a religious rite.*

Bathing and deep breathing are regarded by the Hindus as religious duties, but this does not result in their being shunned by others. We must make a clear distinction between things technically religious and things which, being good in themselves, are for that reason included by some people in their daily religious duties, and which are therefore only apparently religious.

Rules of health have nothing to do with dogma or with blind religious faith.

We should like also to address a special word to those who hesitate to launch out on any course of exercises at all. It is a cause for constant wonder to discover the enormous number of people of all nations who creep through life, with a growing mountain of aches and pains on their shoulders, never making the slightest physical exertion in case they might 'hurt themselves,' or even 'die of heart-failure'!

God made us all alike in fundamentals, with the same simple human needs underneath all our infinite diversities of personality. And one of these simple human needs is exercise—the daily airing and use of all the cells in our bodies, which, for want of this, atrophy and die. Dead cells in a living organism are, as we do not need to emphasize, no help to that organism.

Let us assure these alarmists who have forgotten what it is like to feel the joy and radiance of youthful movement that, if they began slowly and proceeded gradually but persistently, they would within a month or six weeks be astonished to realize that they can, at the age of forty-five or sixty or seventy or even eighty, feel once more the surge of the clear, rapid blood of youth in their veins.

But, these fear-ridden people will say: 'Look at the professional athletes and strong men and women who die of all sorts of diseases, and, moreover, die young.'

We reply that none of these evils is due to any system of exercise. Take, for example, the simple case of the Indian *pahilwan* or wrestler.

Most *pahilwans* are obsessed with the notion that he who can do five hundred *dands* or *jors* is necessarily stronger and healthier than he who can do only four hundred, though the latter may be much the stronger and healthier of the two.

Dominated by this wrong idea, the *pahilwan* always seeks to develop his muscular system at the expense of his vital capacity, and as a necessary and natural consequence, he suffers either from heart-affections or from muscle-binding.

Another example of the *pahilwan's* logic is that the more food he can eat the stronger and healthier he will be. While youth and vigour continue, his faulty logic may appear quite convincing, but when age comes on and forces upon him the wisdom of reducing his exercise, he still goes on stuffing himself, with the necessary and natural consequence of indigestion.

Instances of harmful effects from exercise are mostly due to over-exertion, over-eating, wrong eating, or to other devitalizing excesses.

It is this passion for excess that is responsible for the ills from which the *pahilwan*—and many an ordinary person as well—suffers in later life. Exercise has nothing to do with it.

Excess, not athletics, kills the athlete.

Surya Namaskars have many advantages over the usual types of exercise.

All games, whether eastern or western, require one or more companions. Even the great Indian game of wrestling needs an opponent, while most other games need either many players or various accessories.

Exercise with Indian clubs or dumb-bells cannot be done without clubs or dumb-bells. For riding, you need a horse or a bicycle. You cannot swim without water. Walking, though requiring no apparatus nor a companion, takes a lot of time. A walk of eight or ten miles cannot ordinarily be done in less than two hours or two and a half, at the rate of fifteen or twenty minutes a mile. And almost all out-door exercises depend on favourable weather.

A team-game requires a spacious ground, which may not always be available. In large towns there are not always sufficient playgrounds to accommodate all school, college, and university students. Take Poona as an example of an Indian city. It has over ten thousand pupils attending municipal schools alone, with but four playgrounds for them all, each ground affording space for only two or three hundred children at the most.

The ideal exercise should develop not only the limbs, muscles, and internal organs of the body, but should also promote mental and spiritual development. To make such a physical exercise universally popular and acceptable there should be no necessity for apparatus or appliances; it should be easy to do; it should take a short time to perform; it should be of such a nature as to enable it to be carried out anywhere and by anybody; and should not necessitate a partner or companion. Surya Namaskars fulfil all these requirements.

Moreover, they make for all-round development,

with special tonic effect on the three principal working parts of the body, on the proper functioning of which all health depends. We have found by actual experience that Surya Namaskars, if regularly and methodically performed, render these three organs capable of resisting disease or disease-germs:

(1) *The digestive organs, including stomach, liver, intestines, etc.* An appalling number of people suffer from stomachic and intestinal disorders, such as dyspepsia and constipation. These result in liver trouble, dropsy, piles, diabetes, and a host of other diseases.

(2) *Heart and lungs.* Colds, coughs, asthma, tuberculosis, palpitations and other complaints are symptoms of heart and lung derangement.

(3) *The nervous system, including the brain and spinal cord.* Brain affection is indicated by headache, brain-fag, loss of memory, insanity. Ailments of the spinal cord are paralysis, myelitis, sclerosis, fatigue after slight exertion, depression, cold hands and feet, disturbed sleep.

Surya Namaskars have a particularly notable effect on the nervous system, where resides chiefly the spring of human power. It is from here that energy is transmitted to the tissues and organs of the body. A personality is made strong, compelling, and active not so much by muscle as by the vital energy behind the muscle.

Surya Namaskars directly stimulate the nerve-centres, acting on them in a dramatic and almost visible way, as we shall try to prove in a later chapter.

Children from eight to twelve, with normal health, should do from twenty-five to fifty Surya Namaskars daily; boys and girls from twelve to sixteen should do generally from fifty to a hundred. We have observed that in some schools and colleges physical training, such as gymnastics, drill, etc., is given to students twice or three times per week. Such spasmodic efforts will never produce the desired benefits which we all want every boy and girl to possess.

Persons above sixteen should gradually increase the number of Surya Namaskars up to three hundred daily, according to their capacity. After sixty-five or seventy, however, one should do till death as many as one's bodily condition will allow.

To do about a thousand Namaskars a day for a few months and then to come down to about twenty-five, or to give them up altogether, is positively harmful, in the same way as it would be both foolish and dangerous to eat two or three times the usual quantity of food and then to give up eating altogether. The rules that govern diet and pastime apply to exercise as well. An exercise to be beneficial, should be taken daily, regularly, continuously, and proportionately to one's strength.

To gain the desired end, therefore, Surya Namaskars must be done systematically. They are not a rope-dancer's antics. They must be so performed as to develop and strengthen every part of the body alike.

The reward which awaits those who perform Surya Namaskars according to our instructions will be the constant joy in life which God intended for all His creatures.

To be free from worry or tiredness and to keep healthy and fit for years together without an ailment, without even a slight cold, is a supreme happiness. Once it is known, it is never relinquished at any price.

We must in this preliminary chapter draw attention also to the vital importance of speech in connection with Surya Namaskars. The body is not completely functioning if the vocal cords are left silent. Moreover, the vocal cords when vibrating extend their influence beyond themselves to every corner of the body.

In India the Vedic hymns and names of the sun are recited by Hindus when performing the

Surya Namaskars. To non-Hindus who on religious grounds might object to reciting the hymns, or who might consider that to repeat the names of the sun such as Mitraya Namah, Ravaye Namah, would smack of idolatry, we recommend the use of the meaningless monosyllables, *om*, *hram*, *hrim*, *hrum*, *hraim*, *hraum*, *hrah*, known as *mantras*.

These sounds possess an inherent health-giving virtue, and are too valuable in their physical effects on the body to omit, whatever the religious faith of the performer.

CHAPTER III

THE PRELIMINARIES

In the form in which we present them we believe Surya Namaskars to be the perfect instrument, not only for keeping the body fit, but for warding off old age and disease, invigorating the mind, strengthening the character and will, and increasing to its fullest limit one's capacity for joyous living.

But before you begin we must give you a few warnings and hints.

First, and most important, consult your doctor about your general condition. This is to make sure that you are fit to take any exercise at all, and to enable you to measure your improvement six months hence.

Secondly, though these exercises may look almost absurdly simple, they are extremely difficult to perfect. Unless you have been taking your 'daily dozen' regularly, it will be at least a month before you are ready to put all the ten positions together into a single cycle or Namaskar.

Thirdly, do not forget that one of the finest and most effective little combinations of whistle and red light with which Nature always danger-signals unthinking human beings is *fatigue*. Yet we often disregard this warning and plunge bull-headedly along the road of danger—which is the chief reason why thousands of persons are living on the border-line of physical and nervous collapse.

Every physical exercise should therefore be so taken that, with five to ten minutes' rest after finishing it, one should feel fresh, invigorated, and cheerful afterwards.

In other words, exercise only within the limit of one's strength. Be careful at the beginning, and add gradually to the length of the exercise period as one's strength increases. This golden rule applies most particularly to Surya Namaskars.

Five or ten minutes a day, preferably before breakfast, will be ample for the first few weeks, until you get yourself limbered up. A certain amount of discouragement is inevitable at the beginning of all reconstructive systems of physical culture. That period must be lived through perseveringly if success is to be won. But if you will only stick to it, you will feel so full of new hope in a month's time that you will never want to give up the exercises that have bestowed this new life upon you.

If you wish to prove to yourself by actual

facts how much good Surya Namaskars can do you, have yourself weighed and measured and keep the record in a small book. Put down your weight and the following measurements: height, chest deflated and expanded, waist, hips, thigh, calf, upper arm, forearm, waist, ankle.

Take your weight and measurements again at regular intervals of six months. You will note an astonishing difference. Your weight will become normal, your chest will fill out, your waist and hips will be more slender. Whatever part of you is too thin or too fat will be automatically regulated to its proper size and weight.

Another preliminary, at your own discretion, is to have a piece of cloth, twenty-two inches square, of woollen, silk, cotton, or linen material, of whatever colour and texture pleases you, to place your hands on while you go through the exercises. If your floor is polished lino, a square of rubber would be best, to avoid slipping.

The hands will be placed flat on this cloth and remain there fixed in the same spot for all positions except the standing ones.

To aid concentration, which is a very important part of Surya Namaskars, have a picture of something or someone of significance to you hung up on the wall before you. Or on a piece of cardboard paint a sun or a star or a circle in a vivid colour or colours and put that up in front of you, so that by fixing your eyes on it you will gradually acquire the power of concentrating your mind.

The mind wields such a power in every human action that nothing can be done satisfactorily without it. Therefore, each performance of the Surya Namaskars should be permeated with the active consciousness that one is being helped by them. Concentrate on the idea that every movement is bettering a particular muscle or part of the body, and let all your mind-force and will-power radiate towards that spot. Conceive that the special part is getting stronger, firmer, better-shaped, more active, or thinner, or fatter, and the object will be attained in a surprisingly short time.

The full development of every part, the amelioration of disease, or the removal of pain, cannot be brought about unless the whole weight of mind and will are brought to bear upon the part throughout the exercise.

In this way one begins to establish mental control over one's body, a vital principle in the life of the happy creative man or woman.

CHAPTER IV

BREATH IS LIFE

IT is also advisable, before beginning to learn the exercises, to learn how to breathe. Breathing is difficult to learn for those who have never really breathed since they were small children. Some never take a deep breath except once a year, while on holiday, and then only a few.

There are ten positions in each Namaskar, each following the other in an unbroken rhythm to make a single Namaskar. But remember that the tenth position is a return to the first position, so that it is also the beginning of the second Namaskar. We explain this here because many are confused over the number of breaths taken for each Namaskar.

There are three full breaths—three full inhalations, three holdings of the breath, and three complete exhalations—to each Namaskar. When doing a 'round' of twenty-five, the fourth breath, taken in at the tenth position, is the first breath in the first position of the next Namaskar.

Rhythmic breathing is one of the secrets of

the wonderful power of the exercises to revitalize the body. You may, for practice, breathe rhythmically anywhere you happen to be—standing, walking, or sitting.

The significance of the 'breath of life' has been known since the earliest ages in the East. This knowledge has never been lost, but it has been handed down through untold generations. Recently, the West seems to have discovered the profound truth that air is the elixir of life, and that one of the most precious sources of health, efficiency, and happiness costs nothing.

It is medically ascertained that we take twenty thousand respirations in twenty-four hours. That is, we each have twenty thousand chances to drink deep of the elixir of life. How many of us do so? Watch yourself breathe. You take niggling little sips which fill only a very few of the lung cells. Try taking great deep draughts of air. It is the greatest tonic ever prescribed by any doctor.

Without the breathing, Surya Namaskars would lose half or more of their virtue. They would act like a smouldering rather than a clearly burning fire, like the sun under a heavy cloud rather than in a bright blue sky.

But first you must become aware of your breath. You cannot drink deep of a healing draught that you do not know is there.

Study your breathing. Probably your chest-wall scarcely moves with the intake of air, because it is so small in quantity. Most likely your abdomen does not move at all.

If you try to breathe deep, your chest and shoulders will lift, and your abdomen will be drawn in. This is the wrong way.

Try instead to take the air first into the bottom of the lungs, letting your abdomen expand to its fullest extent; open your ribs like a fan, and lift your chest last of all, without raising the shoulders. You will be amazed to find how much your lungs can really take in.

Now try holding your breath for a few seconds. This may make you dizzy at first. But do not be afraid; it only means that you are so unused to the 'heady' effect of the elixir of life that a good drink of it is too much for you.

As the air is held in the lung cells, it keeps their walls stretched, exercising them and making them strong. As they strengthen, they will expand to air automatically, thus helping you in your effort to breathe correctly.

When after anything from three to sixty or more seconds you exhale, do so completely, making an aspirate sound such as *huh* at the end to ensure that the last particle of used air has been breathed out to make room for fresh air. Exhalation is every bit as important as inhalation.

Now for a warning. All new things should at the beginning be done gently and gradually. You will adjust yourself without discomfort to the new way of breathing if you do so bit by bit. Your lungs, ribs, and chest may ache at first. This will be Nature's way of telling you that you are driving your poor feeble 'bellows to the flame of life' too hard. They have not been used for years and they must strengthen before they can blow the flame into a bright, steady, joyous glow.

The best 'tune' for your rhythmic breathing is seven-time. Count seven for each breath, making the tempo quick at first, and later lengthening it. Fill your lungs in two counts, hold the breath for four, and empty them in one.

We do not suggest that you always breathe in seven-time. If you do so for a total of thirty minutes a day, it will be enough to tune up the rest of your breathing. The more you breathe rhythmically the easier you will find it to breathe correctly at all times, whether you are aware of breathing or not.

It will give you a wonderful sensation of self-control and self-awareness when you can match the rhythm of your breathing with the rhythm of the exercises. You will feel rhythmic all over, and in accord with the great rhythm of life and the universe.

You will be aware of the wonder of living, and of your power to share in it, as no amount of actual adventurous life in the external world can teach you. You will know more about yourself than years of jungle-hunting or dealing with international affairs, big business or worldly success would ever give you. You will feel: 'I can do great things. I can and will live to the utmost capacity that God intended me to.' You will, in fact, be meeting yourself for the first time.

One further point before we come to the exercises themselves. The East and West differ in the manner of exhalation, though this is not a very important distinction. We personally advocate strongly exhalation as well as inhalation through the nose only. It is generally the custom in the West to inhale through the nose and exhale through the mouth. Do which ever suits you best.

CHAPTER V

THE TEN POINTS

We give what is in fundamentals the age-old method of performing Surya Namaskars, and the one followed by our revered father, the late Rajah of Aundh. For fifty-five years he did these Surya Namaskars. We follow the same method, but have developed and changed it in accordance with modern science over a course of nearly thirty years' practice and experiment by ourself in person.

Now, having learned to breathe, you are ready to try the Ten-Point Way to Health. But you need not worry about regulating and controlling your breathing until you can, with practice, do the movements correctly, almost automatically. Then you will find it easy to manage your breath.

Positions are illustrated at the end of the book.

Position One

Spread cloth on floor. Wear as little clothing as possible, the less the better. Let that little be loose and airy. Stand in the sunlight if there is any, with feet and knees together and toes touching the edge of the cloth. Join hands resting on chest and press the palms firmly together.

Raise chest and pull abdomen in and up as far as possible. This stomach movement, pulling in and up and relaxing, is one of the most important in the whole cycle, and is repeated many times. It not only reduces an unsightly bulge, but makes stomach and bowels function properly.

Stand so that a plummet line dropped from the top of your head should go through shoulder, hip, knee, and ankle.

This is the stance taught by the ancient Yogis of India, and is the stance which is being taught to thousands of school children in Great Britain to-day in accordance with the Board of Education's most recent syllabus.

Thus is the wisdom of the ages rediscovered in time of need.

Now, stiffen your whole body, beginning with the feet. Push them into the floor as if you were taking root there. Stiffen especially your waist at the back. You will have trouble in stiffening the stomach flat if it is heavy and enlarged, but in time you will be surprised to find how easily you can control it. The first signs will be that you feel the middle of your spine move back, and the base move forward. Make your spine as straight as possible, especially at the waist, without raising the shoulders.

It is well to begin the stiffening process with the toes and move gradually up to the top of the head, concentrating on each separate part that is being stiffened, doing it slowly and deliberately.

You will thus become aware of every muscle in your body. Proceed from the shoulder to the tips of the fingers, thinking your way to each separate tip, stiffening joint by joint of each separate finger.

Inhale as you do so, and hold the breath. This is Breath One.

When you come to your face, smile gently, lifting its muscles into happy lines.

With eyes fixed on the picture or drawing on the wall, concentrate on the thought of the good that is being done you. Think of the life-giving fresh air reaching lung cells that have nearly dried up for want of it, of your stretched spine energizing the spinal cord and the nerve-centres in your brain, of your taut abdominal muscles rousing the colon to action, your heart sending blood like a mountain torrent instead of a sluggish backwater to all parts of your system.

People with round shoulders or a stoop will feel an appreciable strain in the back. But by proceeding carefully, they should be able in a few weeks' time to straighten out without too much effort, and the poor 'poker spine' will become the flexible instrument which Nature intended it to be.

The sensation you should have is of 'feeling tall,' and it should remain with you throughout the day.

Whenever you feel a strain in doing any of the movements, it would be wise to return for the time being to Position One and do this only for a few days, breathing in seven-time as you hold the position, and concentrate.

Position Two

Keeping the knees straight, drop your hands to the floor, placing them flat upon the cloth just within the edge. As you do so, exhale completely, expelling every last atom of used air. This is the end of Breath One. If your hands do not reach much below your ankles at first, do not be depressed. In a few weeks' time, with regular practice every morning, you should be able to get the palms down. Until then, bend your knees to get your palms down. But aim at straightening the knees as soon as possible.

The palms should be placed almost parallel to the sides of the cloth or at an inward angle of about twenty-two degrees. Some prefer a forty-five degrees angle, while others place the palms with fingers turned in at a right angle to the body. Whatever be the angle, the balls of the thumbs should be on a line with the toes.

In bending, touch or try to touch the knees with the forehead or nose. Squeezing in the abdomen will help to attain this position as well as to expel all the used air.

Do not confuse this position with the familiar exercise of 'touching the toes.' It is much more purposeful and stirring. Thousands who 'touch their toes' religiously every day have no idea what real exercise is like! How many people, after touching their toes, feel the healthy sweat coming from every pore?

Throw your head down as a fisherman flings his bait into a stream. Aim your head at your knees, and turn your eyes upwards towards your waist. This will in time make your spine beautifully supple and as elastic as a child's.

Again, do not overdo this at first, or you will strain your back and limp for a while, and this may put you off the exercises for good.

Unless you are in prime condition, you will also feel dizzy at first. It will do you no harm, however, and only goes to prove how badly balanced you are.

A good plan is to try knitting Positions One and Two together with a kind of pumping rhythm until movement and breathing follows in a single even flow—down-up, down-up, down-up, out-in, out-in, out-in. You will now feel the first sense of rhythmical well-being, as if your nerves had suddenly 'tuned-in' to the peaceful rhythm of the world of natural things like the stars, the tides, the changing of the seasons.

You will find that in Position Two the muscles of the calves, the rear part of the thighs, hips, waist, and almost all muscles of the back and spine receive a strain, which means the gradual development of these parts and the elimination of uric acid and other toxins—the seeds of premature decay and decline.

The spine in this position is stretched—a fundamentally important action. The animals know the wisdom of this. Watch your cat or dog; it stretches its spine a dozen times a day.

Position Three

Your hands are still on the cloth, where they should remain as fixed as roots until you take Position Ten, which is the same as Position One. Try to feel your hands rooted, as were your feet in Position One. They are now your pivot.

Inhale deeply and hold your breath. This is Breath Two. Without bending the arms, drop to your right knee, and lift the head as high as you can, looking upwards. Touch the floor with knee and toes, the other knee jutting ahead of the vertical arm. Press thigh as hard as possible into the side. Keep holding Breath Two.

Drop on the right knee in the first round, on the left in the second, and so on alternatively, each time pressing the thigh firmly into the side.

In this way the left thigh exerts pressure on the spleen, and the right thigh on the liver.

If the liver is out of order, it is advisable that the right thigh only be taken forward until the liver becomes normal again. Those whose liver complaint is hereditary or chronic had better take forward the right thigh always until all signs of their complaint have disappeared.

Similarly, those who suffer from complaints of the spleen are advised to bring forward the left thigh until they find an improvement in their condition.

The fact that Position Two is assumed after a deep breath has the special merit of compressing the lower part of the lungs, thereby driving the fresh air to the upper part of the lungs and thoroughly ventilating the remotest corners, where tuberculosis bacilli generally find a place. This exercise also compresses the spine, and thus there is a special virtue in stretching it in other positions.

Position Four

Still holding Breath Two, and keeping arms and hands as before, raise your body and push leg which has been pressing against side to join the other one. Bend your head into the neck.

Your body should form an inverted V. You will know you have the right position when the muscles behind knees and ankles feel as if they were going to crack. Do not at first try to force your heels on to the floor or you will lame yourself. Wait until all sense of undue strain in the muscles and ligaments behind knee and ankle is eliminated.

By now you will be feeling the existence of muscles of which you were never before aware. The great advantage of Surya Namaskars is that they reach all sorts of small and obscure parts of the body, tuning them all into harmony.

Position Four is particularly beneficial to those with thick or inflexible ankles. The stretching and compressing of the muscles melt away fat and make the ankle light and supple in movement.

Position Five

Keeping hands rooted, drop flat on the floor, touching forehead, nose, chest, knees, toes, but not the hips or abdomen. Try to press the chin in and down against the collar-bone. Exhale Breath Two while dropping, pushing the last remnant out of the lungs with the movement of drawing in and up the abdomen.

The chief aim of Position Five is to lift the abdomen and hips as high off the floor as possible. This squeezes every fraction of useless fat off, leaving the muscles clean and supple.

The bending of the head exercises the muscles of neck and throat, filling out the skin and preventing the 'ropy' or 'crêpey' effect so common in older women.

We find it better to keep the nose also clear of the ground. This intensifies the action on the neck muscles.

The whole of the body above the knees is supported by hands, wrists, and forearms. This strengthens and limbers up the joints, especially those of the wrist, and gives flexibility and graceful movement.

Position Six

Keep hands, toes, and knees as in Five. Straighten arms, inhale (Breath Three), throw chest out as far as possible, curve the back, and look at ceiling, stretching neck back to its fullest extent. Hold the breath.

In this posture practically the whole weight of the body is carried by the arms. Hence they are gradually rendered shapely, strong, and supple. The chest becomes wider and deeper. The bust in women is improved and developed, becoming firm and elastic. In nursing mothers this posture has been known to increase the quantity of milk. As in Position Five, the throat is filled out and improved. Any tendency towards tonsillitis and other throat troubles is checked by this exercise.

Position Seven

You are still holding Breath Three, which is the last and longest breath in the cycle of ten positions, and is held until you exhale it in Position Nine. Rising from Nine to Ten, you take in Breath Four, which counts as Breath One of the second cycle.

Beginning with Seven, the cycle is now completed by repeating the first four positions in their reverse order.

Position Seven	=	Position Four
Position Eight	=	Position Three
Position Nine	=	Position Two
Position Ten	=	Position One

To achieve balance, there is one slight variation. In Eight, instead of kneeling on the right knee, kneel on the left, that is, if you are in normal health. If, as explained earlier, you suffer from liver or spleen trouble, continue to use the same knee.

The table given below will help you at first to memorize positions and breaths. Copy it out, paste it on cardboard, and keep it where you can see it easily.

(1) Stand (in)
(2) Double over (out)
(3) Right leg back (in)
(4) Inverted V (hold)
(5) Flat on floor (out)
(6) Trunk raised on arms (in)
(7) Inverted V (hold)
(8) Left leg back (hold)
(9) Double over (out)
(10) Stand (in)

A single Surya Namaskar, or one complete cycle of ten positions, can be done by an expert in twenty seconds.

We recommend for the beginner fifteen Namaskars in five minutes as an aim. In six months you should be doing about forty Namaskars in ten minutes.

Above all, do not be in a hurry. Take your ten minutes a day without fail, as regularly as you catch the train to town every morning. Put your whole heart and mind into it. Know that if you persist, seeming miracles will happen to you. Work at the different positions separately, putting together first those that come most easily to you. One day you will suddenly find yourself going through the entire cycle automatically, and you will be rewarded with a glorious sense of freedom, power, and happiness.

CHAPTER VI

VALUE TO WOMEN

As we strongly recommend Surya Namaskars for women—young and old, maids and matrons (even pregnant women or nursing mothers)—the following instructions, based on actual experience, will be found useful to womenfolk in special conditions.

The Namaskar exercise should be suspended during the menstrual period, from the time the menses actually begin to flow until they stop, the normal period being four to six days. At the end of the period the exercise should be begun again without delay.

An expectant mother may continue the Namaskar exercises as usual until she completes the fourth month of pregnancy. From the fifth month to the end of the seventh the exercise should be modified in accordance with her state of health. If she is in any doubt, she should consult her doctor. From the beginning of the eighth month until child-birth she should only do the deep breathing and reciting of the *mantras*. The *mantras* are explained fully in Chapters XI and XII.

Even after the suspension of the Namaskars, no pregnant woman should sit or lie down in laziness, but should do light and pleasant work, such as domestic duties, walking, gardening, and so on until the very hour of child-birth.

Resumption of the exercises after child-birth should be undertaken on the advice of the doctor. Some women could do them safely and with great advantage within a month of child-birth. Others would have to wait several months. In any case, they should be resumed gradually, care being taken to avoid all strain or tiredness.

Whenever a girl or woman cannot take, or is prevented from taking, any bodily exercise for reasons other than ailment or disease, she will be helped by reciting the *mantras*, concentrating her mind as strongly as possible on any desire she wishes to attain.

Apart from the above special conditions, women should follow exactly the same rules that govern men in performing Surya Namaskars.

To those who hold that women do not need as much exercise as men it should be pointed out that woman—the mother—is, in the words of an Indian poet, 'the mine of heroes and great men,' and that you cannot expect a weak and sickly mother to bear healthy, strong, and long-lived children.

Are the present generation of our young girls and women models of physical perfection?

Is it not a fact that in many cases they come of parents who have rarely enjoyed normal health?

Is it not a fact that many young women are averse to marriage because of the duties of motherhood?

Is it not a fact that there is a general dread of motherhood in the minds of young wives throughout the world?

Is it not a fact that there is an appalling infant mortality amongst our city-dwellers?

Is it not a fact that very few young mothers are able to suckle their children and that the widely advertised 'foods' have to be depended upon mainly because the mother is often a mother when she is hardly fit to be one?

In his novel, *The Silver Spoon*, John Galsworthy described a modern young woman as 'flat as a board behind and before.' This still holds true of the vast majority of young women from China to Peru.

The only remedy for this most deplorable state of things is to put our girls and women through a scientifically designed course of physical culture. There is no doubt at all that girls and young women derive benefit from Surya

Namaskars. Indeed, cases are known of matrons of fifty who only after a short course have almost regained their youth.

To those readers who can afford it we recommend at least a cursory perusal of numerous magazines and books on physical culture that have recently been published in India, Europe, and America, and of the large output of literature about the science of eugenics. All who study these carefully will be convinced that the same course of physical training as is prescribed for men is also beneficial for women—with, of course, a few minor adaptations.

Girls and women in great numbers have benefited from Surya Namaskars in bodily and mental health and in general appearance. We vouch for this personally.

It might be of interest to know what Surya Namaskars have done for our Ranisahib.

Before she took up the exercises eleven years ago, she had backache whenever she worked for an hour or so in a sitting position. Now, though she studies and works harder and longer in the same position, she feels no pain whatsoever. It has entirely disappeared.

She used to suffer occasionally from indigestion and constipation. These ailments too have disappeared. Pain above the waist used to afflict her, but that has ceased. A number of menstrual irregularities have also cleared up since she began these exercises.

Weakness subsequent to child-birth disappears more rapidly than before, and parturition is practically painless. Our children are healthier and stronger. The Ranisahib looks younger, though she is the mother of eight children.

Even more convincing is the case of Mrs Saubhagyavati Sitabai Kirloskar, wife of the tutor to the Ranisahib. She is now aged sixty-one and is the mother of ten children.

Within six months of beginning to do Surya Namaskars systematically, most of the superfluous fat from which she had suffered for many years and all her rheumatism and backache disappeared. Her digestive system began to function better, her hair stopped falling out and its former lustre returned; her complexion became clearer and ruddier, even her nails showing a redder tint. Perspiration lost its unwholesome odour—an awkward personal complaint from which she had suffered much. The muscles of her arms, legs, and bust became firmer and stronger. Her chest measurement increased by two inches, while that of the abdomen decreased by two inches.

Surya Namaskars have a peculiar importance

for women in so far as they more than men depend upon physical attractiveness, and by the harmonious action of these exercises in toning up all their physical processes they acquire a very bloom of personality.

CHAPTER VII

WARDING OFF OLD AGE

PREMATURE old age and premature death are tragedies. The spirit of youth is always and everywhere desirable, nay, absolutely necessary. It is well said that 'it is better to wear out than to rust out.' An old man or woman, though taking exercise, may not be quite as springy or nimble as a youth or a maiden, nor should one expect to have a 'twenty-five face on a seventy-five body'; but discontinuance of all bodily activities will invariably bring about rapid degeneration and decay.

The following conditions, among others, are universally regarded as indispensable for 'making old bodies young':

(1) *A strong, straight, and flexible spine.* A straight spine is one that enables you to carry your body erect. The central nervous system consists of brain and spinal cord with nerve ramifications radiating throughout the body. It is the spinal cord that represents life. If it is diseased, death will follow; if it is unhealthy, the body will be unhealthy. If the nervous system is not functioning normally, all the involuntary actions of

the heart, stomach, liver, kidneys, and glands will fail to work properly.

(2) *A strong back.* A man is as strong as his back. Since most old people are seen with their backs bent, it is generally thought that a curved back and rounded shoulders are inevitable in one's decline. This is, however, wrong. With proper care and regular exercise all men and women not deformed from birth can carry themselves like true soldiers of life to the very end.

(3) *A strong stomach.* After the age of about fifty-five or sixty a man or woman should have only one meal, or at most two, in twenty-four hours. Overeating, wrong eating, or taking stimulants and drugs, results in the accumulation of undigested food in the colon, and this is one of the contributory causes of constipation, which 'mothers a brood of diseases.'

(4) *Colon cleanliness.* Most people are likely to conclude that because their bowels move once a day, they are therefore free from constipation. But how they move is the question. You must, therefore, get your colon examined and see that it is neither encrusted nor engorged.

(5) *Flexibility of Joints.* A majority of old folk suffer from stiff joints—joints affected with rheumatism or gout, as a result of overeating or wrong eating. A joint in any mechanism, whether of

wood, steel, or flesh, will function stiffly or not at all if neglected.

(6) *Absence of Obesity.* It has been found that obesity tends to shorten life. If you wish for active longevity, the girth of your abdomen must be considerably less than that of your chest.

(7) *Active skin.* It is not generally recognized that the greatest single excretory organ is the skin, upon the proper functioning of which the health to a large extent depends. No real reason exists for loading ourselves with a burden of unnecessary clothing in our country, or in any country, for that matter. At a conservative estimate clothes must be responsible for more than ten to fifteen per cent of disease and for a considerable portion of the cost of living. Daily exposure to fresh air and sun will render the skin active and young.

(8) *Youthful spirit.* 'A man is as old as he feels' is an adage that is applied with greater force to those of advanced age. The minute a man loses faith in his youthful spirit and begins to feel like an old man and adopts the manner of an old man, he will rapidly become old. Faith is the dominant principle in man.

As soon as a person retires from his usual service or work, he thinks that he is old and has nothing to do in the world but to spend the rest of his life in laziness, under the groundless apprehension that any bodily activity or exertion will shorten his life. But he should remember that it is rusting out and *not* wearing out that causes premature senility and death.

Youthful spirit depends upon the activity of body and mind. Bodily activity and mental activity are interdependent. Therefore, be inoculated with the feeling that you will ever continue young and active, and you will remain young and active.

Mental activity is necessary to the best degree of health—and especially in old age. It is found from statistics that professional men and mental workers, such as scientists, philosophers, theologians, etc., live longer than manual workers and those given to hard bodily labour.

If you want your mind and body to function normally, they must both have regular occupation or exercise.

It is but natural for man to wish for a long life and youthful spirit. But many, instead of obeying the wise laws of Nature, waste their time, money, and energy in the vain search for some panacea, not realizing that it is only to be found in their own bodies. The mad craze for countless specifics, patent medicines, and drugs in order to prolong life only shortens it in the end.

There are men who have reached old age after a clean, plain, useful, and strenuous life, and to such it is suggested that they submit themselves to a moderate course of Surya Namaskars in order that their useful and active life may be prolonged.

There is another class of old men on whom senility is forced by misfortune in the shape of compulsory residence in crowded cities, sickness, bereavement, or other reverses in life: to such Surya Namaskars are useful in that they minister not only to the body but to the spirit as well.

The third class of prematurely old men consists of those who have played ducks and drakes with their health and youth and have thoroughly ruined their constitutions, being in consequence given up by doctors. Even to these can be held out a promise of redemption, if they be like children and follow faithfully the practice of Surya Namaskars.

It has been said that man begins to die the moment he is born. The inevitable end, however, can be postponed for a long, long time, if only by proper exercise we rid ourselves of the products of decay. If we ever really learn to do this, we should, barring accidents, live far beyond the limit of one hundred years.

CHAPTER VIII

USE IN SCHOOLS

WE have been fortunate enough to convince our people at Aundh of the usefulness of physical education in general and of the Surya Namaskars in particular, and they have taken to them with such enthusiasm as to demand a state regulation to make Surya Namaskars compulsory in all the schools.

It is our dearest wish that the students of our schools should extend the benefits of the system not only to their families, but to all with whom they come in contact.

Should our dream be realized, there will be seen within the short space of five or ten years a vast improvement in the health, strength, and spirit of those who attend school and college. We will not, however, be fully satisfied if the health of our boys only is improved, because Society requires that the health of our girls—the mothers of the race—should be improved even before that of the boys.

One of the chief merits of Surya Namaskars is that it can be adapted to group or mass exercise. Under proper supervision, hundreds of students—boys and girls—can be made to take this exercise simultaneously, thus affording the double advantage of efficiency and economy of time. The students may be grouped according to age, height, or capacity.

We are convinced from our experience of group exercises performed in all the primary and middle schools as well as in the high school of the Aundh State for the past twelve years, that Surya Namaskars are the ideal exercise for use in large groups.

It is hardly necessary to observe that the daily practice of Surya Namaskars, far from interfering with any game or pastime requiring physical exertion, actually adds to the enjoyment of it.

We are not opposed to outdoor games, sports, or gymnastics. Far from it! The main point we want to emphasize is that, combined with the pursuit of any sport or game, there must be a daily exercise like Surya Namaskars, which can be done singly or *en masse* all the year round in order to lay a real and lasting foundation of health and strength. For this exercise puts one in condition to take part in any sport or athletics requiring strength and endurance.

A systematic daily performance of Surya Namaskars forms a basis for all other bodily activities, because it is found to give in a marked degree the power of control over body and mind and the capacity to use one's strength to the best advantage in games and sports, especially those which require prolonged exertion, without injurious results. It minimizes the risk of overstrain, especially of the heart.

Normal all-round health, acquired by the daily performance of Surya Namaskars, will enable children to render a better account of themselves not only in any sport or game but in everyday life as well.

The experience of two schoolmasters bears out what we have said. We give their own account below.

The Experience of Mr Shankar Hari Javadekar, Head Master, Marathi School, Indapur, Poona District

In the month of May 1925, stomach ache began to afflict me daily at about two o'clock in the afternoon. The pain gradually increased to such a pitch that despite the varied treatment of doctors and physicians at Indapur, I felt as though several scorpions were stinging me in the stomach. Then I went to Poona, where I placed myself under the treatment of a well-known medical practitioner for ten days. There was slight relief, but the pain persisted.

I returned home to Indapur and continued to take medicine and follow a regimen as prescribed by the Poona doctor, but all in vain. The thought that the disease might permanently sap my energy and constitution had taken the heart out of me, when the book on Surya Namaskars by the Chief of Aundh came to hand. A careful perusal of the book induced me to try the Namaskar exercise for relief. I did try and was able to do fifty Namaskars within a week, as I had already done a great deal of gymnastic work.

The wonderful alleviation of my disease, brought about by the exercise within so short a time, encouraged me to continue. I gradually increased the number of Namaskars to two hundred, when all pain vanished and I was restored to health. I was very happy to find that Surya Namaskars achieved what all medical treatments and other exercises failed to do. I have since then been a staunch adherent of Surya Namaskars.

Having been thus convinced of the therapeutic and prophylactic value of the Namaskar exercise, I wished that all my assistant teachers and pupils should also profit by practising this wonderfully efficient exercise.

I accordingly convened a public meeting, consisting of teachers, students, and a large number of townsfolk, and delivered a lecture on the necessity and importance of Surya Namaskars for keeping one always fit and healthy. The lecture proved so effective that all the teachers and students agreed with one voice to do the Namaskars in the school every day during school time. The public, too, were so favourably impressed that they immediately subscribed towards a fund necessary to erect a spacious and convenient hall for doing this exercise.

The hall was soon built to the delight of us all. As many as a hundred and fifty students are now taking this Namaskar exercise simultaneously in this hall under my direction.

Another idea soon struck me: I wished to find by actual comparison if Jors and Baithaks, systems of Indian gymnastics, if daily and methodically practised, would produce the same results. I therefore made two batches, each consisting of twenty-five boys of almost the same age, strength, stature, and circumstances. Their individual measurements and weights were recorded in a register specially kept for the purpose, before each batch commenced its own form of exercise.

The same period of time was allotted to both the parties to do their respective exercises. Twelve months' regular practice conducted under my personal supervision proved the decided superiority of Surya Namaskars over Jors and Baithaks.

The Experience of Mr G. K. Gokhale, M.A., Superintendent, New English School, Hubli, Dharwar District

Having decided to give a trial to Surya Namaskars I came to Aundh from Hubli and put myself in the hands of an expert in Surya Namaskars, who is also a great enthusiast. I took my first lesson on the 13th October 1928, and it required four or five days for me to learn the movements. I was doing only half a dozen Namaskars daily as my body was stiff and the various muscles were put to a considerable strain in doing even such a small number of Namaskars. But gradually they appeared easier to do and in a few days I could complete twelve Namaskars almost according to the rules laid down. I could increase by about six Namaskars every half week or so. To my great surprise, on the seventeenth day of my training, I could do fifty Namaskars without being particularly fatigued or feeling out of breath. This I consider to be a great merit of the *mantras* and hymns, which are so graduated that the period of rest due to their recitation goes on lengthening as the Namaskars go on increasing in number. If the length of the *mantras* for the first twelve Namaskars be supposed to be one unit the length of the *mantras* for the next six Namaskars is two units; for the next three Namaskars, it is four units, and for the next three it is twelve units; so that you feel quite fresh by the time you have finished the first cycle of twenty-four or twenty-five Namaskars.

I can assure all those who may be thinking of taking this Namaskar exercise that it is easy to learn and quite safe, as it does not put any undue strain or do any injury to any muscles or organs of the body. To do the movements exactly according to the rules prescribed would involve such a strain, but the beginner is not expected to aim so high; it is better for him to attain perfection gradually. In fact, some of the positions are so hard that they can only be done perfectly after months of practice.

Even with the little practice I have had I am beginning to feel the beneficial effects of the exercise. The extra fat on my abdomen is vanishing and my chest seems to be expanding. The constipative tendency, which had so far appeared natural and inseparable from me, seems within control, and I am feeling more buoyant and energetic.

CHAPTER IX

OUR OWN EXPERIENCE

WHEN young we studied wrestling under Imam Uddin, a well-known professional wrestler from the Punjab. We also practised Jor, Baithaks, and Indian clubs, but, in accordance with the accepted doctrines of the old school of wrestlers, we used to eat unnecessarily fatty foods, and thus put on an excessive amount of fat.

In 1897 we read about Sandow, a famous physical culturist. We purchased all his apparatus and books, and for fully ten years practised regularly and continuously according to his instructions, with the result that the chest measurement remained the same, while that of the waist and abdomen showed a marked reduction. Since 1908, being influenced by the example and advice of our esteemed friend Shrimant Sir Gangadharrao, Chief of Miraj, we have been doing Surya Namaskars every day with *mantras* and Vedic hymns, and the result has been a most remarkable lightness of body, buoyancy of mind, and a general feeling of youthfulness, which must be experienced to be understood.

But the highest benefit of all is that during the

past twenty-one years, we have been absolutely free from fevers and other ailments, and have never even suffered from a cold or cough, which is regarded as inevitable even by medical men. But the most surprising proof of the stamina and resisting power of the body acquired through Surya Namaskars lies in the fact that, though we submitted to plague inoculation no less than four times, we had no fever and experienced no sort of muscular pain sufficient to prevent us from doing our daily Namaskars.

We submit that this twenty-seven years' experience and study have qualified us to state with a measure of authority that of all the systems of physical exercise, Surya Namaskars stand first and foremost in promoting bodily and mental health and in endowing one with an equanimity of mind, which remains unruffled even under the most trying conditions.

In the circumstances, it may be of interest to know the daily programme which at the age when most men 'sit about' in a kind of mental and bodily torpor, we follow with all the vigour and joy of youth.

We rise each day at 3.30, with a sense of welcome for the work before us. Until 6.15 the time is spent in bathing, exercising, and morning worship. Exercise includes an hour's Surya

Namaskars and a brisk climb up a hill six hundred feet high.

Our schedule then proceeds more or less as follows:

6.15–7.30. Breakfast with Ranisahib and children.
7.30–9.30. State affairs.
9.30–10.30. Painting while listening to the reading of newspapers.
10.30–11.30. Dinner.
11.30–12.30. Reading.
12.30–1.30. Siesta.
1.30–3. Literary work.
3–6. Official work. Correspondence, disposing of petitions, examining routine work of the secretaries, superintending sculptural, block-making, and other works, and so on.
6–6.30. Evening worship.
6.30–7.30. Evening meal.
7.30–8.30. Reading to the Ranisahib and children.
8.30–3.30. Sleep, which comes within five minutes of resting the head on the pillow, and is sound and dreamless.

This has been our diet for many years, and was worked out after persistent trial:

Breakfast. Two cups of cow's milk, warm and fresh from the udder, and a little cream mixed with honey.

Dinner. About eight ounces of boiled whole brown rice (rice with hull only removed and not pearled or polished); between two and four ounces of whole-wheat bread; a little pulse, one or two raw or cooked vegetables without condiments; a little milk or milk products, such as curds, butter-milk, ghee; fruit and nuts.

Supper. The same as dinner, but much less in quantity.

All fried articles are generally excluded from our dietary.

We drink fresh, cool, spring water, scented with some fragrant flower, as rose or jasmine. We never drink water at meals but always an hour after meals, and whenever we feel thirsty between meals.

Many ignorantly think that if a sufficient quantity of beverages other than water be consumed, water as such may be dispensed with. There could be no greater fallacy. It must be emphasized that from a therapeutic point of view there is no substitute for pure water.

We eat nothing between meals, not even fruit. All stimulants and narcotics, such as tea, coffee, cocoa, tobacco, and so on, are absolutely avoided.

In addition to regular daily exercise and a wholesome frugal diet of vital foods, we practise frequent fasting—complete or partial.

CHAPTER X

EVOLUTION OF SURYA NAMASKARS

We are often asked the question: 'Has the method of Surya Namaskars which you are now advocating been followed by you from the beginning?'

In reply, we shall try briefly to show how the present system was gradually evolved from the old method.

It was in 1908 that we first began to do Surya Namaskars in the old style. According to this the knees were not straightened while bending over, nor was the foot brought forward on a line with the palms, and it was not necessary to stand erect at the beginning of each Namaskar or to regulate the breathing in the way we have indicated.

After doing the Namaskars in this way for about a year, we tried one day to bring the toes of one leg forward on a line with the palms, and found that it put a greater strain on the abdomen and waist. This was the first improvement made on the old style.

On another occasion, while attempting to straighten the knees when bending over to place the palms on the ground, we experienced a still greater stretching sensation in the calves, thighs, waist, abdomen, and throughout the back. A material improvement resulted.

Following the custom of the old school of wrestling and athletics, we ate freely of fatty and proteinaceous foods, such as cream, butter, and nuts, and consequently put on an excess of fat all over the body, especially round the abdomen. As we felt it necessary to reduce the girth of the abdomen, all such movements as gave a vigorous stretch and compression to the abdomen were gradually introduced.

The changes thus made in the mode of doing Namaskars vigorously strained and acted upon the stomach and abdomen muscles, and gradually got rid of a tendency to constipation. Though the bowels sometimes fail to function the first thing in the morning, they do open freely an hour or so after the Namaskars.

When required to stand for a longer time than usual in order to recite certain prayers and hymns, we tried to stand erect, with chest inflated and thrown forward, and felt an appreciable strain in the abdomen and waist regions. Since then we assumed this attitude in *every* Namaskar.

When taking the right foot forward, a studied

pressure on the right side of the stomach, and a similar pressure on the left side in taking the left foot forward, were found to stimulate the liver and spleen respectively.

With the introduction of these improvements, we naturally stopped the old way of doing four or five Namaskars in one breath. Discovering as well that a complete exhalation greatly facilitated the action of pulling up the abdomen, we made use of this in the positions of bending over and touching the ground with chest and forehead.

At first we began to take one full breath for one Namaskar. Finally, we found it most useful to accompany each drawing-in of the stomach with a complete exhalation, so that three full breaths came at length to be included in performing a single Namaskar.

We have explained this at some length, because we feel that we have played our small part in helping our fellow-men and in helping to change matters.

CHAPTER XI

HEALTH THROUGH SPEECH

We now come to a part which will seem obscure, and perhaps even childish and forbidding, to many western readers. Do not hurry to read and ponder over this chapter. Take your time with the exercises alone, and there will come a moment when you will be prepared to understand what we have to say here sympathetically, and without prejudice due to preconceived ideas. Then perhaps you will try the additional help of speech in connection with the exercises.

Indian thinkers and healers have known for countless generations the secret of gaining health through speaking, and have brought it to a fine art. The amazing thing is that it has not been more universally recognized that the vocal cords are a part of the body which need exercise as much as any other part. Why leave them dead and silent while all the rest of the body is being tuned up?

Any one who has studied singing will know what joy and invigoration, as well as self-control, come through singing, and in what good condition it tends to keep the throat and chest.

The natural thing for the man or woman going about the tasks of the field and home is to whistle or sing.

Millions of our Indian people have experienced the wonderfully healing and vitalizing powers, physiological as well as psychic, possessed by the apparently meaningless sound *om*, known time out of mind as the Pranava, and of the six sounds *hram*, *hrim*, *hrum*, *hraim*, *hraum*, and *hrah*, known as the Bija Mantras.

The loud and clear repeating of these seven sounds influences the vital organs such as the heart, stomach, and brain, and serve not only as a prophylactic (preventive) but as a therapeutic (curative) as well.

The first sound *om* is pronounced with a prolonged 'o' and a prolonged 'm,' rhyming with 'home.'

Next comes *hram*. In this all the sounds are long. The correct pronunciation is *hraaammm*, rhyming with 'calm.' The aspirate sound 'h' proceeds from the heart. Every time, therefore, you say *hram*, the heart vibrates vigorously. The process of purifying the blood takes place in the heart, for the pure blood that runs to any affected part of the body is pumped out by the heart. If that blood is made pure before it reaches the affected or diseased part of the system, then only the desired result will follow, i.e. the cure of the affection or malady. Should impure or toxic blood circulate through the body the affected or diseased part is likely to get worse instead of being cured. Every *mantra*, therefore, is made to sound with the initial aspirate 'h' with a view to vibrating and strengthening the heart so that it pumps out pure blood only.

Just as each *mantra* begins with the aspirate 'h' it ends with the labial nasal 'm.' Every normal respiration has to be made through the nose. It is this respiration that also helps to purify the blood. The oxygen taken in with each inhalation comes in contact with the veinous blood and renders it pure and red, and the carbon dioxide from the impure blood is breathed out. As respiration is done through the nose and windpipe, both of these organs should be kept free from ailment or disease. Each *mantra* is made to terminate in the continuous or prolonged nasal 'mmmm' to vibrate and keep healthy the nose and windpipe.

Likewise in each *mantra* there stands the lingual 'r' between the initial aspirate 'h' and the final nasal 'm.' The consonant 'r' is held almost as important as *om*. In uttering the consonant 'r' the tip of the tongue strikes the front palate and tends to vibrate the brain. Hence the proper utterance of the psychic syllables *hram*, *hrim*, etc., vibrates and invigorates the heart, windpipe, and brain—three of the vital organs, the soundness of which is necessary to keep the system strong and healthy.

In reciting the *mantras* one has to open the mouth for 'h' and to shut it for 'm.'

There is an elegant couplet in Sanskrit eulogizing *hram* which when freely translated means: 'The mere utterance of "ra" in *hram* drives out sin-toxin from the open mouth, and being afraid of its re-entrance, the consonant "m" serves the purpose of a door by closing the lips.'

The continuous long vowel 'a' in *hram* strengthens the ribs, purges the alimentary canal of toxins, drives away lethargy, and cleanses the upper portion of the lungs by stimulating them. The *mantra* '*hram*' has proved a curative for asthma, bronchitis, and for predisposition to tuberculosis.

The long vowel sound 'i' in *hrim* (as 'ee' in 'seen') stimulates the action of the throat, palate, nose, and the upper part of the heart. The repetition of *hrim* clears the respiratory and digestive passages of phlegm secreted or collected there. In the first or second round of Namaskars, done with the *mantras*, it is sometimes, if not often, necessary to eject the superfluous mucus from the nose, throat, or mouth, but after about two rounds the respiratory passage is thoroughly cleared.

The long vowel sound 'u' in *hrum* (as 'oo' in 'room'), effectively excites or stimulates the liver, spleen, stomach, and intestines, and reduces the abdomen. Women suffering from chronic disorder of the lower region of the abdomen will immensely profit by repeating *hrum* loudly and fully.

The compound vowel sound of the syllable *hraim* (as 'i' in 'time') stirs up the kidneys. The repeated utterance of *hraim* in the Surya Namaskars serves as a diuretic.

The compound vowel sound of the *mantra* '*hraum*' (as 'ou' in 'round'), acts on the rectum and anus and helps them to function normally.

Last, but not the least, is *hrah*, which vibrates the chest and throat.

Thus all these seemingly meaningless sounds produce vibration in different vital parts of the system, stimulate them, purify the blood, and consequently remove disorders, ailments, and diseases in those regions.

This table will help you to remember the pronunciations of these curative syllables:

om rhymes with 'home'
hram rhymes with 'calm'

hrim rhymes with 'seem'
hrum rhymes with 'room'
hraim rhymes with 'time'
hraum as in 'round'
hrah as in 'hurrah'

These syllables should be repeated loudly and clearly on assuming the first position in each Namaskar.

This is the abbreviated *mantra* chart which we suggest for beginners. It is well to count the Namaskars as well, as indicated:

Namaskar 1. *Om hram* one
2. *Om hrim* two
3. *Om hrum* three
4. *Om hraim* four
5. *Om hraum* five
6. *Om hrah* six
7. *Om hram* seven
8. *Om hrim* eight
9. *Om hrum* nine
10. *Om hraim* ten
11. *Om hraum* eleven
12. *Om hrah* twelve
13. *Om hram hrim* thirteen
14. *Om hrum hraim* fourteen
15. *Om hraum hrah* fifteen
16. *Om hram hrim* sixteen

17. *Om hrum hraim* seventeen
18. *Om hraum hrah* eighteen
19. *Om hram hrim hrum hraim* nineteen
20. *Om hraum hrah hram hrim* twenty
21. *Om hram hrim hrum hraim* twenty-one
22. *Om hraum hrah hram hrim* twenty-two
23. *Om hrum hraim hraum hrah hram* twenty-three
24. *Om hrim hrum hraim hraum hrah* twenty-four.

CHAPTER XII

THE SOUNDS THAT HELP

It will be noticed that the length of the *mantras* is increased towards the end of the round of Namaskars. This is to give longer periods of rest and normal breathing, so that one never gets out of breath no matter how many rounds are done.

As a matter of possible general interest we explain the method used by many of adding to the *mantras* the twelve names of the sun in the Sanskrit language, which gives a further lengthening of the period of rest and further help from the practice of speech.

These names of the sun are:

Mitraya Namah ('friend of all, I bow to thee').
Ravaye Namah ('praised by all, I bow to thee').
Suryaya Namah ('guide of all, I bow to thee').
Bhanave Namah ('bestower of beauty, I bow to thee').
Khagaya Namah ('stimulator of the senses, I bow to thee').
Pushne Namah ('nourisher of life, I bow to thee').

Hiranyagarbhaya Nahma ('promoter of virility, I bow to thee').

Marichaye Nahma ('destroyer of disease, I bow to thee').

Adityaya Nahma ('inspirer of love, I bow to thee').

Savitre Nahma ('begetter of life, I bow to thee').

Arkaya Nahma ('inspirer of awe, I bow to thee').

Bhaskaraya Nahma ('refulgent one, I bow to thee').

The following abridged method of using the names of the sun is suggested as being suitable for Christians, Hindus, non-Hindus, Parsees, Mohammedans, and members of any other faiths alike:

Use *om* once or twice or more with each repetition of sounds.

Precede each name of the sun with one *mantra*, two names of the sun with two *mantras*, four, with four, and twelve with all six *mantras* twice over.

A round accompanied by these vocal exercises will take about eight minutes.

Before closing this chapter, we should like to say a few words on the subject of our ancient learning.

In these days, dominated by machine-made experience, people who have lost confidence in their own creative powers are fond of railing at the ancient culture of their race, whether it be Indian or any other.

Many are swayed by the fallacious argument that had their ancient civilization been good and sound, they would not be reduced to their present deplorable condition.

On the other hand, those who study our ancient heritage and are fully aware of its value seem unable to make their teaching acceptable by presenting it in terms of modern medical and hygienic science.

It took Coué to teach us the virtue of *Japa*, or constant meditation upon a certain idea, or Haddock to instruct us in the importance of will-power, or William James to enlighten us on the significance of mental control. Any one who reads the works of these men even cursorily and compares their teachings with those of ancient Indian sages will not fail to be struck with wonder at the resemblance.

Quite unarmed as they were with the mechanical appliances available to modern science, our sages made many discoveries far in advance of their time.

It may be news to most of our readers to be

told that the catheter is mentioned in the Atharva Veda, the date of which cannot be later than 3000 B.C., and that the surgeons of the time of the Rigveda could fit up a metallic leg to a woman so as to enable her to move about.

The ancient *rishis*, or sages, appear to have known something of higher mathematics also. They were very fond of using a phrase which may be rendered: 'If infinity be subtracted from infinity, the remainder is infinity.'

There is a story in the Puranas that Soma married the twenty-seven daughters of Daksha and that four of them brought forth the four planets —Mars, Mercury, Jupiter, and Venus. The great astronomer Bentley read into these marriages a concealed reference to the conjunction of the Moon with the several planets in those constellations. Bentley's calculations were checked by Hindman, and it may now be asserted that the Puranic story refers to astronomical phenomena which took place within the course of sixteen months about 1424 and 1423 B.C.

We learn from the testimony of Greek historians that at the time of Alexander the Great there were *vaidyas*, or physicians, in the Punjab who could successfully cure cases of snake-bite; these Alexander was perforce compelled to engage when his Macedonian physicians confessed their inability to deal with such cases.

We could give many further examples of ancient Indian truths, which have been independently discovered by modern scientists, but this is hardly the place to do so.

Brahmans have been, rightly or wrongly, charged with deliberate concealment of their wisdom. It is not for me to examine the justice of this charge, but it cannot be too deeply impressed that nothing would give us a greater happiness than to see the entire world enjoying the fruits of our ancient civilization.

CHAPTER XIII

CURE OF CONSTIPATION

We shall devote an entire chapter to the subject of constipation, as we consider it one of the greatest enemies of the human race.

Constipation is a condition in which the evacuations from the bowels are of insufficient frequency and amount, more or less faecal matter being retained in the intestines.

Modern civilization with all its conquest of Nature has miserably failed to confer permanent and lasting health on civilized man.

On the contrary, the incidence of disease is appallingly great.

If one is called upon to express in one word the many and multifarious diseases from which the modern man is suffering, that one word will be 'constipation.'

From constipation start more than ninety per cent of ills, inasmuch as toxins or poisons from waste food matter flood the system and attack you in your weakest point, whatever that happens to be.

Poisons set up by constipation give conditions favourable to cancer and other dread diseases.

But the inroads of constipation are so insidious that the sufferer often ignores them, finding nothing very much out of the ordinary.

There are a thousand and one causes of constipation, practically all of them being preventable or curable. But all this apparent multiplicity of causes can be traced to wrong diet or overeating, and to lack of proper physical exercise.

Few people ever enjoy completely perfect health. You realize it in your own case. How often you feel below par! Not ill, yet not certainly a hundred per cent fit. Science now tells us why this is so. Wrong diet or overfeeding and lack of exercise are the cause.

How shall we change this state of affairs? By drugs? The tendency of people suffering from constipation is to turn to drugs for relief. But drugs tend to perpetuate the ailment instead of removing it. It is in our opinion sheer folly to believe that drugs cure diseases. This belief is in itself a contributing factor to the building of the worst form of constipation.

Proper bodily exercise, combined with a balanced diet, will prevent and cure constipation. As more unhappiness of civilized folk is due to constipation than to any other ailment, it follows that any form of exercise that will prevent and cure constipation will be a priceless boon.

Surya Namaskars are pre-eminently calculated to give those movements to the abdominal muscles and to the entire digestive canal that stimulate the peristaltic action of the bowels, on which alone depends a thorough evacuation of waste matter.

The muscles which are of primary importance, and which are also most apt to be neglected and left unexercised by a normal man or woman of sedentary pursuits, are those of the walls of the abdomen.

Most of the positions in Surya Namaskars are specially designed to give to the abdominal walls those stretching and contracting movements which best secure elimination from the colon. And we want to emphasize this particular feature of Surya Namaskars. In no other form of exercise do we find these systematic stretching and compressing movements.

You will, perhaps, ask: 'Why should I need the Surya Namaskars when I work hard all day with plenty of exercise?' The best answer to this is for you to analyse your own bodily conditions. Remember that the reason you are not in the best of shape physically and mentally is because you do not get the *right* kind of exercise. Surya Namaskars not only normalize the bowel functions but build you *all over*. No daily employment can do this, as all employments at best develop and strengthen some parts of your body at the *sacrifice of others.*

Constipation seemed in our case to be a family complaint passed down from father to son. The ailment ran throughout our family.

Was it only due to a continuation from generation to generation of the same dietetic or hygienic errors? In any case, since we suffered from the complaint while doing systematically and continuously for several years other types of exercises than Surya Namaskars, we were convinced we had to put up with it as a family trait.

This constipation produced piles, which had to be removed by operation about 1909. The removal of the piles gave us great relief, but constipation was still there.

Since we commenced Surya Namaskars, however, constipation—the arch-enemy—gradually diminished until it totally died away within a couple of years. To-day we are quite free from it, though it is a matter of general experience that constipation has a firmer grip in advanced age. We should doubtless be in even more vigorous health to-day if we had taken to Surya Namaskars from boyhood.

CHAPTER XIV

TUBERCULOSIS

We shall give another complete chapter to the second great scourge of mankind—tuberculosis. We use the term in the sense of pulmonary or lung tuberculosis.

The germ-theorists hold that consumption is caused by microscopic germs, called tubercle bacilli, because whenever any part of the body is attacked by tuberculosis vast numbers of these germs are found in it. But at the same time they admit that people with sufficiently strong resisting power *cannot* be affected by these germs. Then it follows that if the resisting power be increased there would be no fear of these bacilli—hence no consumption. An increase in one's disease-resisting power can be attained by Surya Namaskars.

Only when the soil is first prepared upon which the tubercle bacillus can thrive will its depredations become noticeable.

Germs of various kinds, such as those of diphtheria, typhoid, malaria, or tuberculosis, are found in the throats or spittle of healthy persons. The average dweller in a city breathes and swallows millions of disease germs. Some succumb, others resist.

We therefore wish to emphasize with all the power we possess that if you have acquired and retained vigorous health and resisting power by doing Surya Namaskars, you need not be afraid of germs.

It has been estimated that one-fifth of the human race succumb to tuberculosis.

'The greatest brains of the medical profession have sought a specific remedy for years. They still seek it. Humanity waits.'

The habit of sleeping out of doors at night and living out by day does not bring about the results sought for, though it helps considerably to cure and prevent consumption.

The only *infallible* remedy for the cure and prevention of tuberculosis lies in the correct method of breathing.

The expression 'deep breathing' is generally taken to mean filling one's lungs with air with a view to increasing their capacity. But the *secret* of deep breathing is not so much in the method of inhalation as in that of exhalation. The manner of exhalation as expounded by all of our authorities, such as Patanjali, Yajnavalkya, Vasistha, Hata-Yoga-Pradipica, Amrita-Bindu-

Upanishad, and others, is to exhale slowly through the nose only and to press in or squeeze the stomach as far as one can do in order to expel all the toxin-laden air from the lungs.

Most modern American and European authorities on deep breathing agree with our principle and method of exhalation.

'Just consider,' observes Dr W. R. Lucas, 'what deep breathing will do for you. No matter what your physical troubles are, *deep breathing* will help to overcome them. It helps to cure cold feet by bringing more oxygen into the blood. It helps to drive away constipation by giving internal massage to the bowels. It helps to overcome torpid liver by the exercise given to that organ. It helps to cure rheumatism by securing enough oxygen to burn up some of the foreign deposits in various parts of the body. It costs nothing and has only good after-effects.'

The amelioration and cure of consumption and the prevention of pneumonia depend as much on the air you exhale as on the air you inhale.

You will notice how this scientific method of exhalation is adopted in Surya Namaskars. In performing one Namaskar one has to squeeze or pull in the stomach three times to secure complete exhalations.

You thus do automatically as many as seventy-five deep breaths in performing *one* round of twenty-five Namaskars. In four rounds of Namaskars, which an average man or woman can easily do within thirty minutes, you actually complete three hundred deep breaths, i.e. three hundred full inhalations, three hundred holdings of breath, and three hundred complete exhalations!

CHAPTER XV

POINTS ABOUT DIET

THE results of an examination of the opinions of modern American and European dietitians and of the facts of our own personal experience have led us to place great emphasis on the importance of diet. We do not wish, however, to dogmatize on this subject; a few broad suggestions are all we shall attempt to offer.

There should be an ample supply of fresh clean milk in one's daily dietary. Each individual should have at least a cup of milk at each meal. All milk-products—cheese, buttermilk, butter—may be eaten with benefit.

A liberal use of fresh fruits and berries is always desirable. A small quantity of nuts should form part of one's meals.

It is vitally important that with grains the whole natural kernel be used, with husk or bran unremoved, as in whole brown rice (unpolished) and whole wheat. These grains will give better results if they be allowed to germinate a little before being used.

Peas, beans, kidney beans, lentils when slightly

germinated and crushed in a food-chopper, seasoned to taste and mixed with grated coconut and onion, will make a very tasty and substantial food, affording a goodly supply of vitamins and mineral salts.

Fresh fruits are not always available throughout the year, except at very high prices, but whole grains, peas, and the various kinds of beans, especially if germinated, serve to a certain extent the same purpose as fruits.

All leafy vegetables should be eaten whenever possible uncooked, for cooking destroys part of their value.

Potato, carrot, and onion can be used in an infinite variety of ways—boiled, baked, steamed, or raw.

Tomato, a valuable vegetable from the nutritional point of view, is an important article of the dietary; for the tomato yields large quantities of vitamins, and mineral salts.

Eggs or the yolks of eggs are next in importance to milk.

Refined sugar might, with advantage, be dispensed with. It may be used very sparingly when absolutely necessary. Raw sugar or honey is better.

But whatever one eats, one should regulate the amount according to the needs of the body.

A manual worker will consume larger quantities than a clerk.

Water should be drunk freely between meals. A good plan is to drink a large glass of water the first thing in the morning, and several glasses between meals. A famous doctor once said that if all his patients drank, as he did, eight glasses of water a day, none of them would ever again come back to him.

This chapter on diet must include a word of warning, especially to the young enthusiast in health culture. Do not be led away with the idea that the true test of your physical powers is your capacity to gorge large quantities of eatables. Emphasis is laid on this particular form of weakness, because it is so common.

Another form of weakness is the habit of 'bolting.' Both these weaknesses should be avoided. They result in throwing an unwarranted burden on the digestive organs and produce conditions favourable to the inception of disease. Remember that many diseases are due to overeating or hurried eating. A good rule is to eat less, and take more time to eat it.

If you feel that your liver or stomach is not working properly, do not drug yourself, but observe a fast and take the extra load off your stomach or liver.

The question is often asked: 'How many meals a day should be taken?' Though the answer may depend on a number of factors, such as the capacity of the eater, the life he leads, the quality and quantity of the food he takes, we venture to say from our own experience and that of others that for an average man or woman, three meals a day with no snacks between are quite enough. Tea should be a drinking, not an eating, ceremony.

However careful we may be in selecting the proper food and in regulating the quantity, some undesirable and unnecessary edibles and liquids find their way into our stomach, owing partly to our ignorance, and partly to force of habit, and are likely to cause trouble.

To counteract this unpleasant result, fasting, as a remedial measure, is absolutely necessary.

The Golden Rule is to fast when you lose appetite. Loss of appetite is Nature's warning that no more burden should be laid on the digestive organs. It is a good plan to set apart for fasting a certain day each week or each fortnight.

In many religious orders certain fast-days have been set aside, as Lent, Roza, Ekadashi, etc.

A fast may be complete or partial. In a complete fast, nothing but pure water is taken.

For a partial fast try an all-milk diet of milk

diluted with water, or a honey-and-water mixture, or clear soup, or orange juice, or lemon juice, or buttermilk. With the soup, orange, lemon, or buttermilk diet, plenty of water should of course be taken as well.

A word or two on cooking food the health way will not be out of place.

The ordinary methods of cooking vegetables, cereals, and other foods in large quantities of water destroy the nutritive elements contained in them. The excess water after boiling is usually discarded and the washed-out remnants of the food are eaten.

Our cooks and housewives boil dead many vegetables, cereals, and legumes. To make sure there is no life left in them, the water is sometimes changed two or three times! All the mineral salts are lost in this way—salts which are vitally necessary to health.

When the vegetables are thus rendered tasteless and flavourless, sauces and spices are poured over them in the vain effort to restore to them the lost taste or flavour.

These same foods, however, when properly cooked, retain all the nutritive elements and flavour, and have a richness and individuality of taste that could not be equalled or imitated by the most elaborate sauces and dressings.

There are many excellent ways of cooking foods, but the principle underlying all is exactly the same.

In brief, it is: Let steam do the work of cooking.

There are many steamers on the market, at all sorts of prices. One may cook an entire meal in some of them. These waste not a single drop of the goodness in the foodstuff put into them.

One may also 'steam' all kinds of food by putting very little water in the pot, covering it so that it is practically air-tight, and putting over a very low flame.

For example, to cook six medium potatoes, put them in any kind of saucepan of a size to just hold them. Put half a tea-cup of boiling water in, and cover closely. When they are done, the water should have completely evaporated. Potatoes should always be cooked in their jackets to preserve the goodness, being skinned only after cooking.

A little shaking of the pot over the flame should make your potatoes fit for a king—perfectly dry, and full of their own goodness.

Or, if you are using the heat of the oven for baking, put the tightly covered dish with the small amount of water into the oven, and the potatoes or vegetables will cook there just as successfully.

Now that fire-proof glass is so readily obtainable, an excellent idea is to cover the cooking vessels with a fire-proof glass plate. One may then observe the progress of affairs, and tell at once when the water has boiled away, without lifting the cover.

Another word of caution! We are out for health, happiness, efficiency, and longevity, and we are not out for large, prominent muscles. Therefore, we would advise you to find out for yourself the quality and quantity of food that is good for you as well as the amount of exercise, work, recreation, and rest that you need.

One has personally to adjust the equation between work and play, sleep and wakefulness, food and fasting, exercise and rest by careful experimentation. General directions are all that can be given here.

There is a beautiful saying in Marathi which means that men's constitutions differ as their faces, and hence each individual must find out for himself his personal needs.

Proper selection of diet from vital foods, with fasting at regular intervals, when coupled with systematic Surya Namaskars, should in a single generation produce a wonderful improvement in the health, strength, vigour, and bodily size of a people.

CHAPTER XVI

NEW LIFE FOR OLD

THIS chapter will be in the nature of a summary. We shall bring together all the reasons which make Surya Namaskars a universally acceptable, practical, and convenient system of exercise.

They can be taken by all persons without exception.

They can be done singly or in groups of hundreds or thousands.

They can be done outdoors or indoors, day or night, at all seasons of the year.

They take only a few minutes to do.

They are easy to learn and to remember.

They are not special exercises for this or that part of the body, but for the whole body.

They require no outfit.

They can be taken throughout one's life, from childhood to old age, and thus easily become a habit.

They can be taken anywhere at a moment's notice wherever one goes.

They cost nothing and require no initial outlay or upkeep.

They strengthen the entire digestive system and cure or prevent constipation.

They develop the lungs and prevent tuberculosis, and will help to heal it to a great degree.

They invigorate the heart, and will remedy high blood pressure, palpitations, and other derangements by improving the circulation of the blood. Active circulation is a prime law of health.

They tone up the nervous system, doing away with brain-fag, forgetfulness, worry, and other mental troubles. Though shattered nerves take a longer time and are more difficult to repair than other cells, the correct performance of the exercises will slowly but surely restore them to normality.

They stimulate glandular activity and give a new vigour to the glands. Owing to the stretching and compressing movements of the throat, the thyroid gland is stimulated and tendency to goitre is obviated. Correct glandular functioning is vital for health and attractiveness.

They improve the colour and function of the skin by enabling it to eradicate toxic impurities through profuse perspiration and to absorb vital energy from the atmosphere. A clear skin glowing with health and vigour is a winning factor for men and women in business and social life.

They strengthen the neck, shoulders, arms, wrists, fingers, back, waist, abdomen, thighs, knees, calves, and ankles. Strengthening the back is known to be a simple but efficient remedy for kidney troubles.

They improve and develop the bust of maids and matrons; keep it firm and elastic; restore it to normal functioning, and increase the quantity and improve the quality of milk in nursing mothers.

They stimulate the uterus and ovaries; remove menstrual disorders and consequent pain and misery; render child-bearing less painful and less dangerous.

They prevent the hair from falling out and lessen its tendency to greyness.

They counteract the bad effect of high heels, tight shoes, belts, collars, and other restrictive clothing demanded by custom or fashion.

They reduce redundant fat, especially the fat about the abdomen, hips, thighs, neck, and chin.

They reduce the abnormal prominence of

the Adam's apple by the forward bending of the neck.

They destroy the offensive odour of perspiration.

They reduce bow-leggedness.

They make you immune from disease by giving a tremendous increase to your disease-resisting power.

Besides normalizing the functions of the internal organs, they give you external shapeliness, grace, and attractiveness.

They are the quickest method for increasing and maintaining youthful buoyancy. The spirit of youth is an invaluable asset. It is wonderful to know that you are fit and can get the most out of life.

They will generate in you good and optimistic thoughts, and give a charitable and sanguine turn to your disposition.

They will, in short, unlock the door to the glorious health, strength, efficiency, and long life which every man is heir to.

And it will cost you nothing to try them.

Surya Namaskars are capable of giving all these gifts to men and women because they possess the unique feature of co-ordinating the action of all the vital organs, muscles, and other parts of the system, which are thus developed and strengthened simultaneously. We do not profess that the Surya Namaskars are a panacea for all the ills that the human flesh is heir to, but we have no hesitation in assuring our readers, men and women, young and old, rich and poor, strong and weak, that this system of exercise, if loyally and steadfastly followed, will reward the performer with superb health, vibrant energy, and 'new life for old.'

Life is a song of happiness to me and mine through Surya Namaskars. This book is my thank-offering.

PHOTOGRAPHS

I. SURYA NAMASKARS DEMONSTRATED BY AN EXPERT, APPASAHIB, SON OF THE RAJAH OF AUNDH

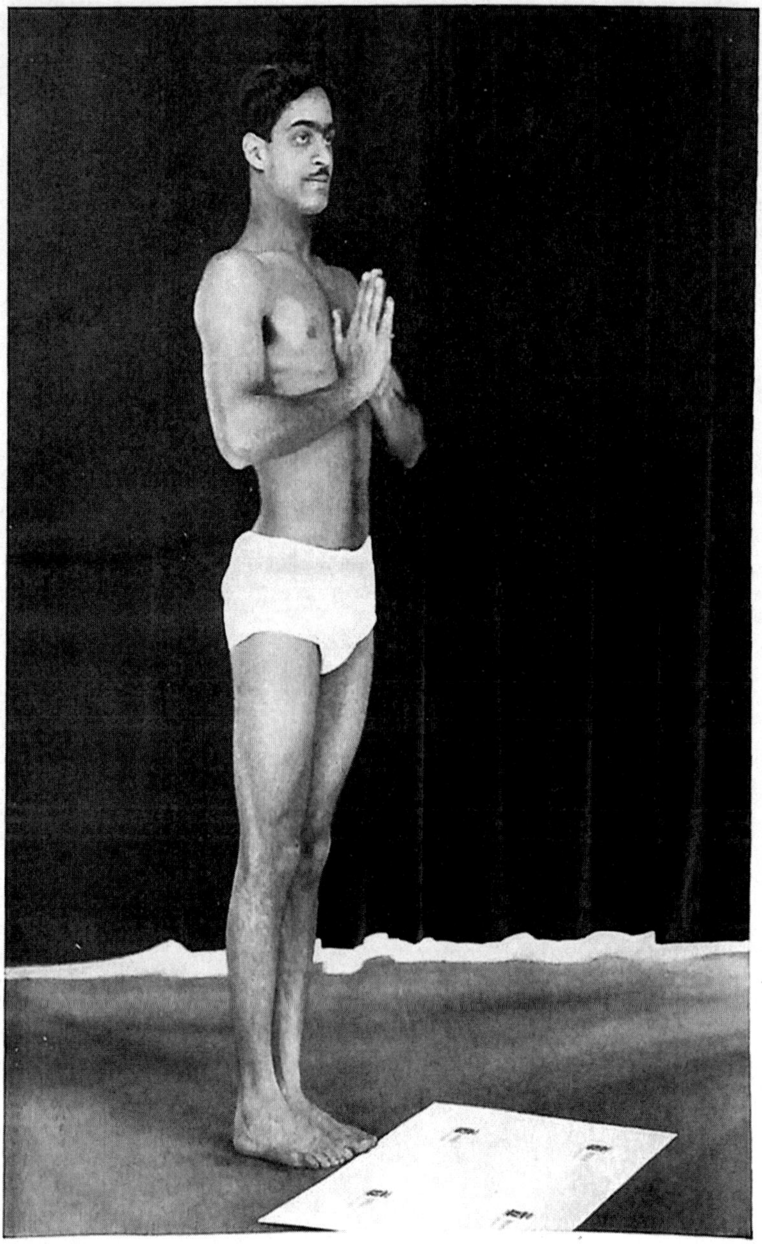

1 Appasahib is here beginning a Namaskar. He is concentrating—a vitally important preliminary.

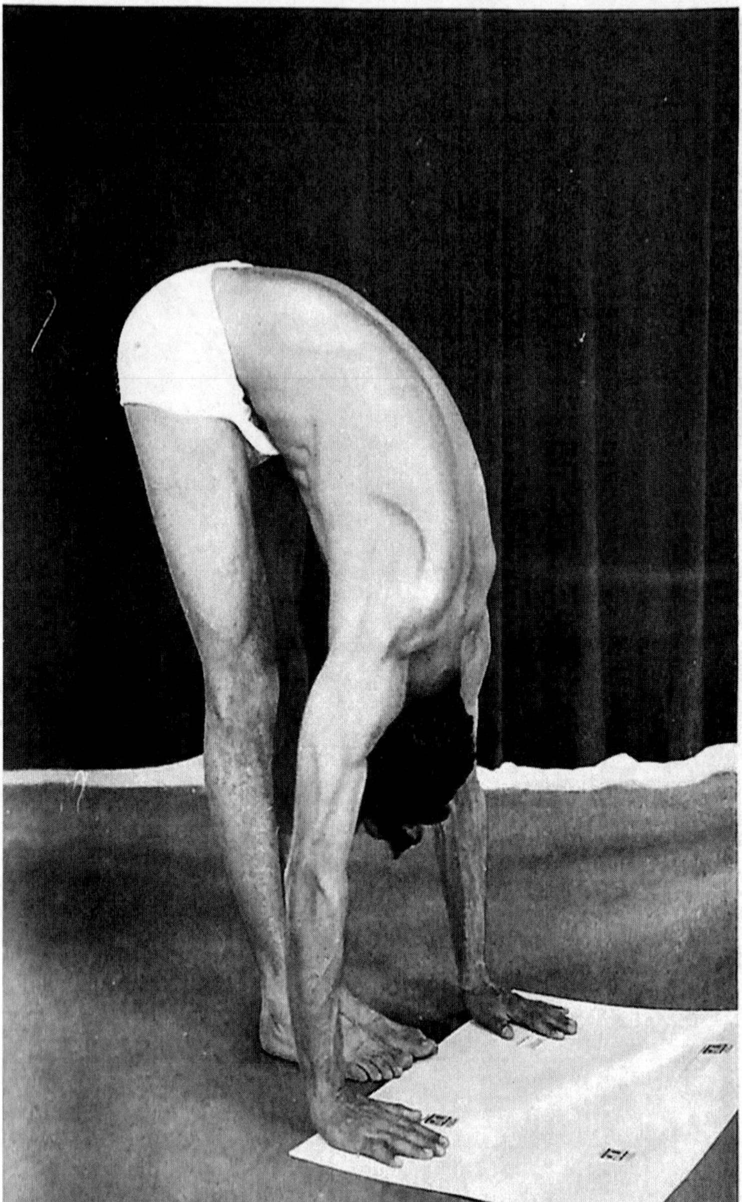

2 Feet remain rooted, knees straight, wrists at edge of cloth in line with toes, and stomach is drawn deeply in.

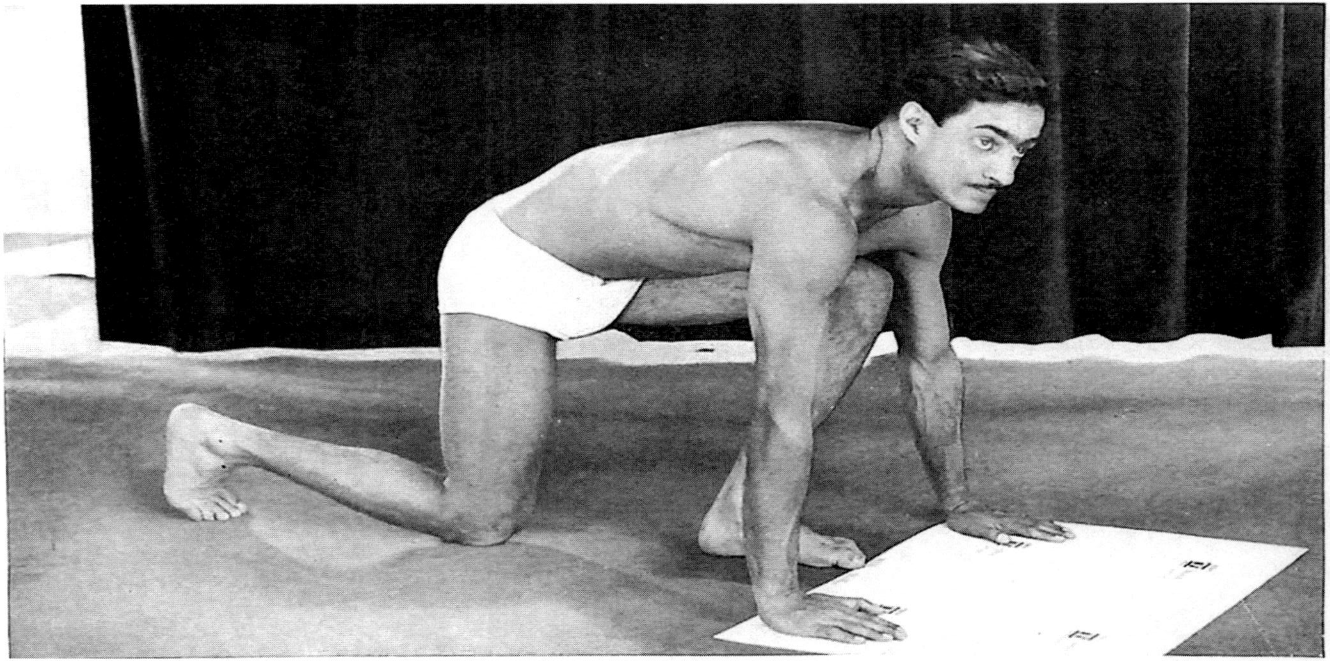

3 One thigh in line with arms, other pressed deep against trunk, and head lifted back as far as possible. The least strenuous position.

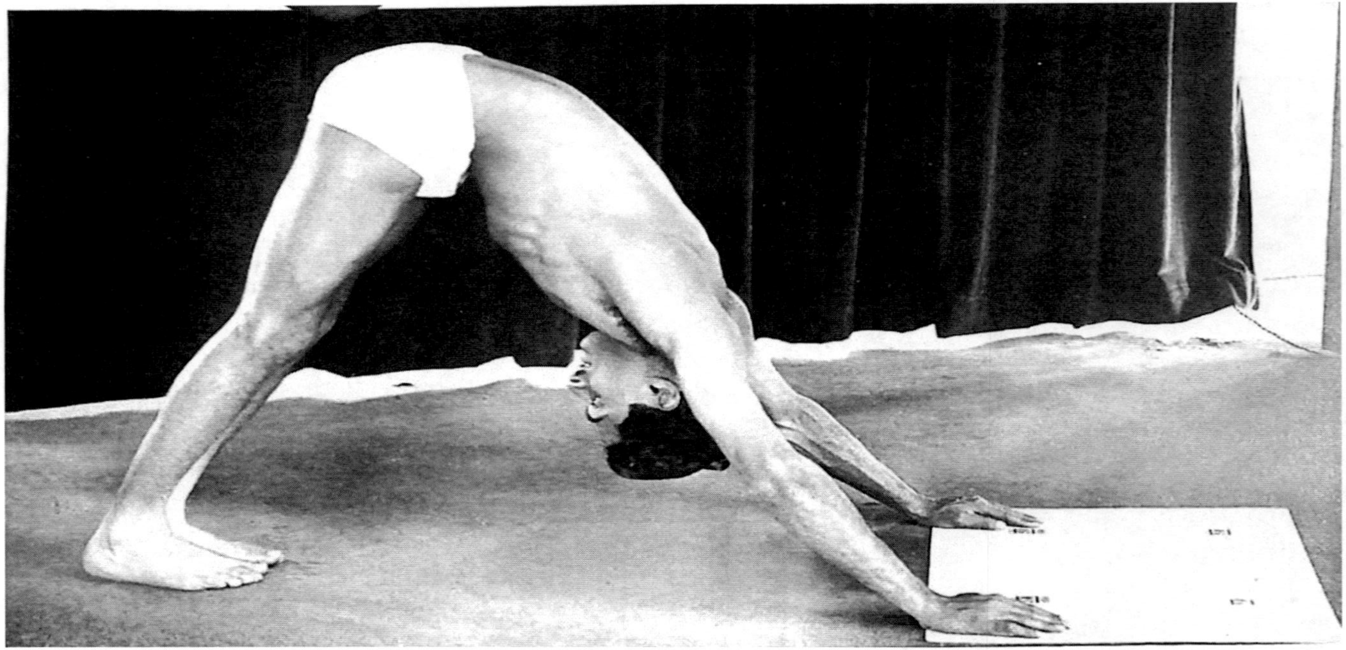

4 Appasahib's heels do not quite touch ground. They should, but he demonstrates under unfamiliar conditions, and is not up to standard.

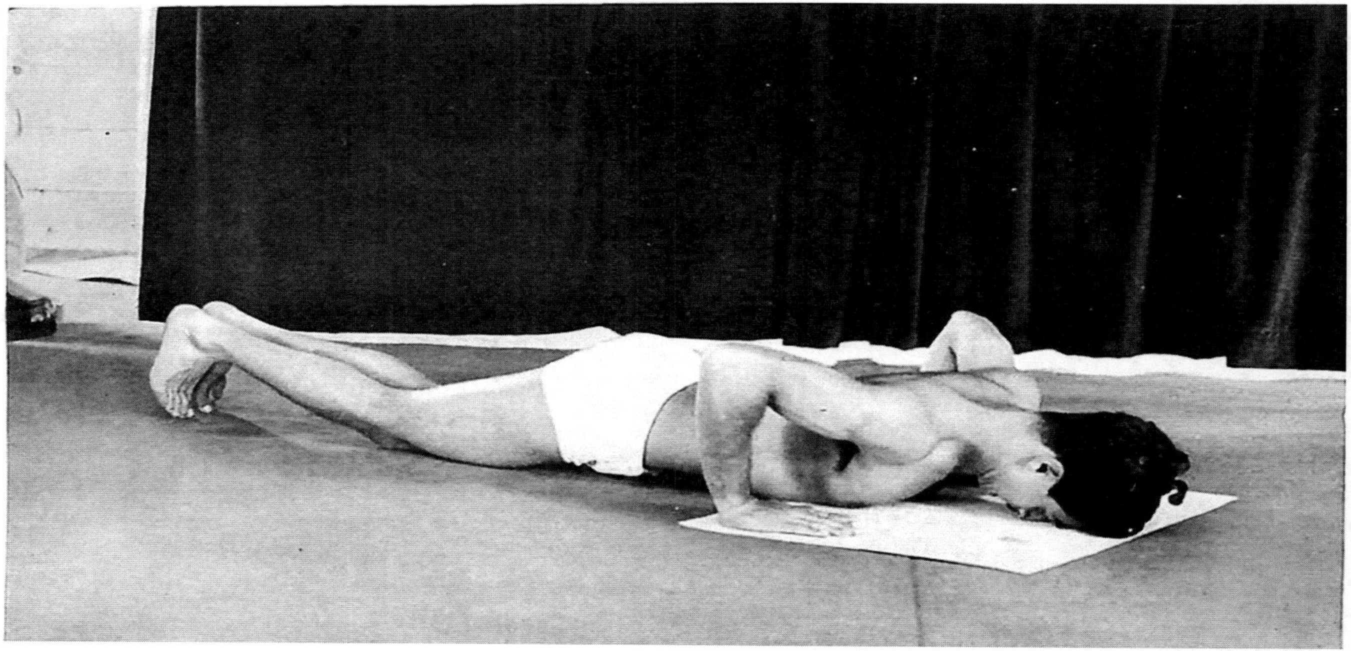

5 Note how high the elbows are raised above trunk. Chin and abdomen are drawn as high as possible from the floor.

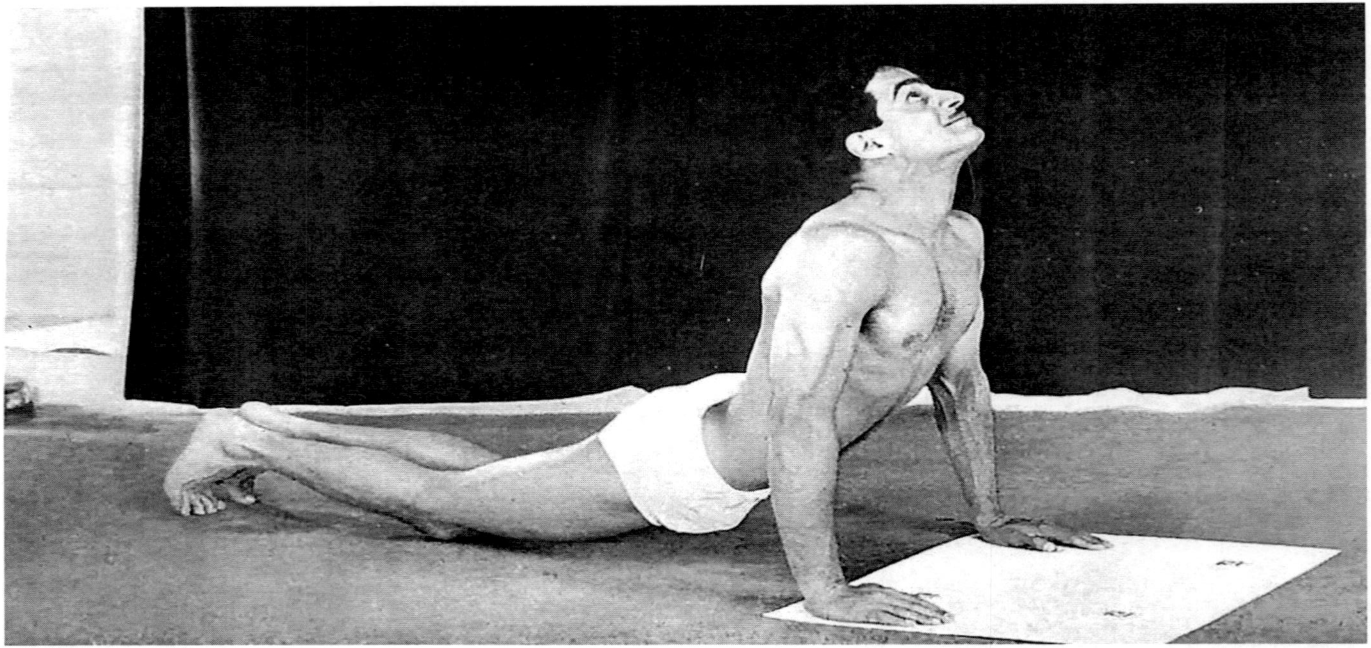

6 Front neck muscles from being compressed expand to their limit, back neck muscles compressed in turn, and chest inflated to capacity.

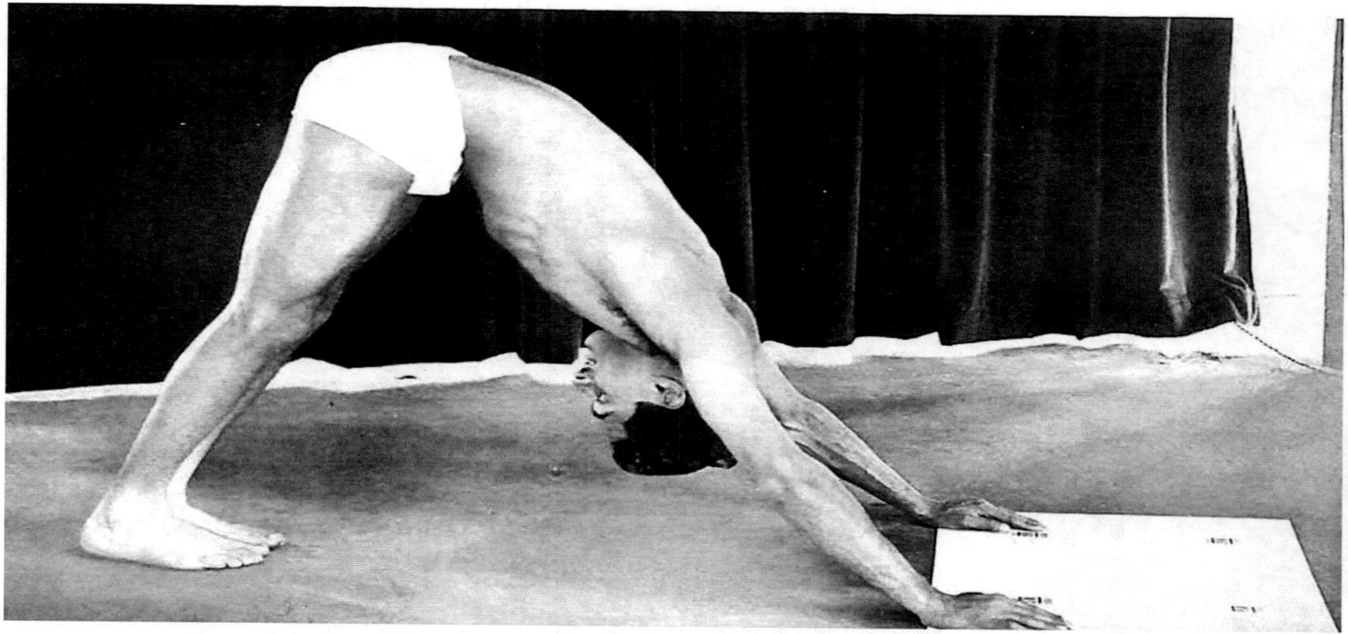

7 Reverse rhythm begins. Reversing brings entirely different muscles into play, and also for flexibility. Head is slightly out of line.

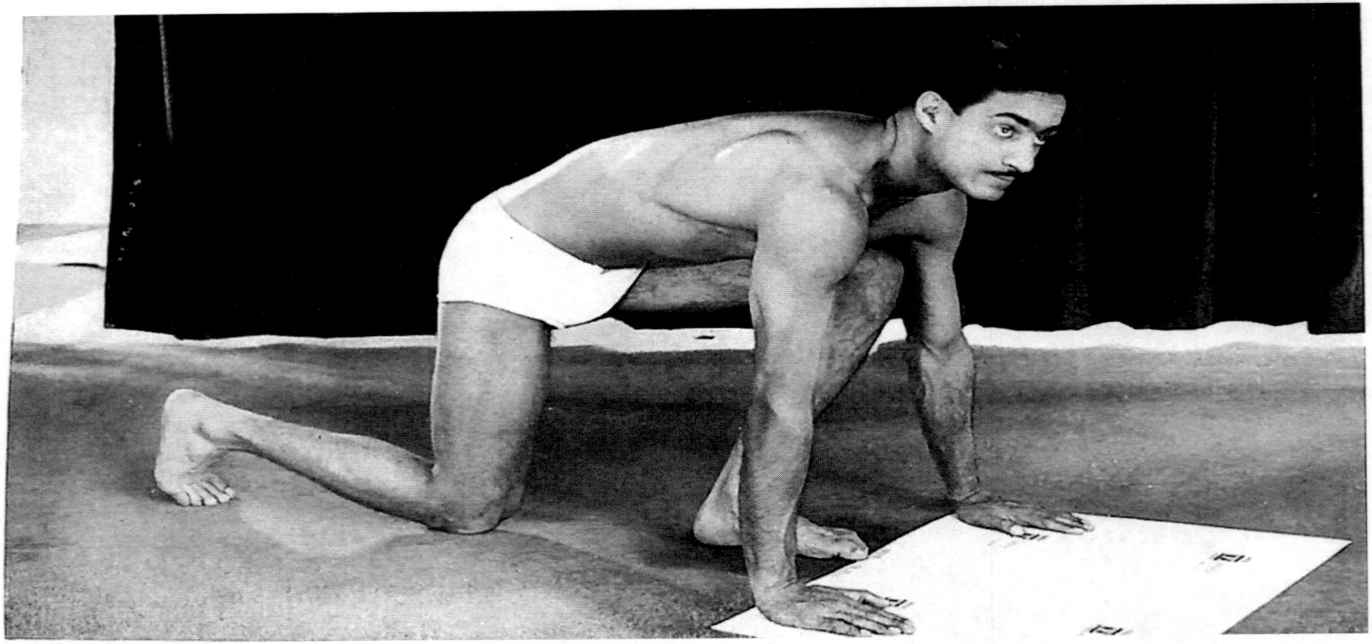

8 Position 3 repeated backwards. For balance, put other foot back. Pressure is then exerted against other side of trunk.

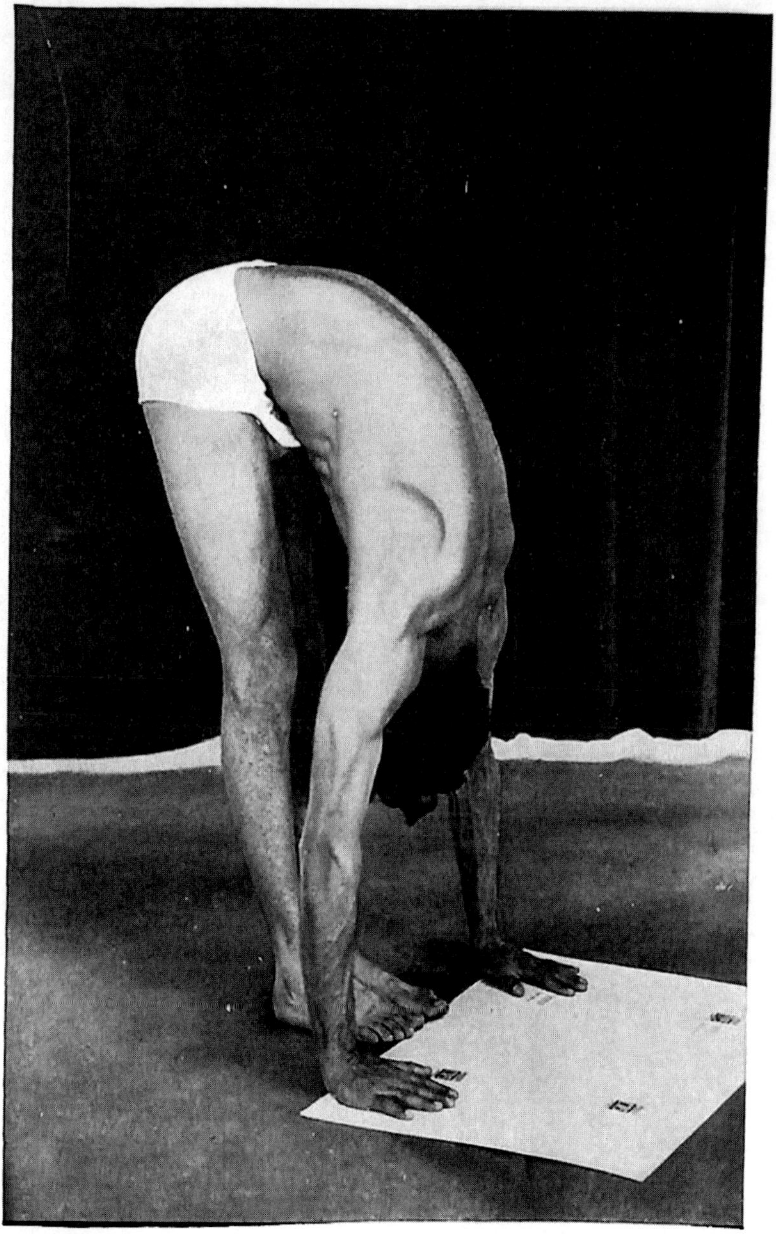

9 Hands kept fixed while raising trunk and straightening legs. The nose should touch the knees.

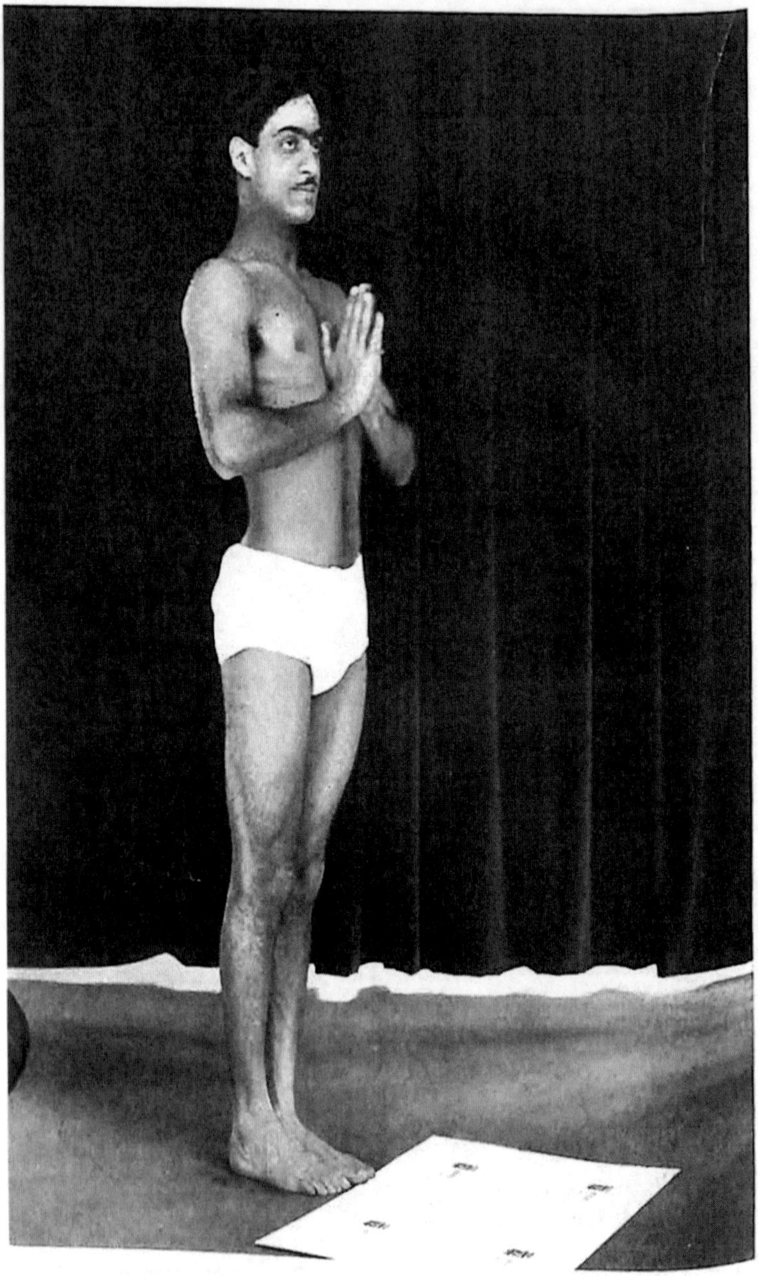

10 The finish and start of a Namaskar. If tired, rest in this position, breathing in 7-time (see page 41).

II. SURYA NAMASKARS DEMONSTRATED BY A LEARNER, MISS RITA BRYNTESON

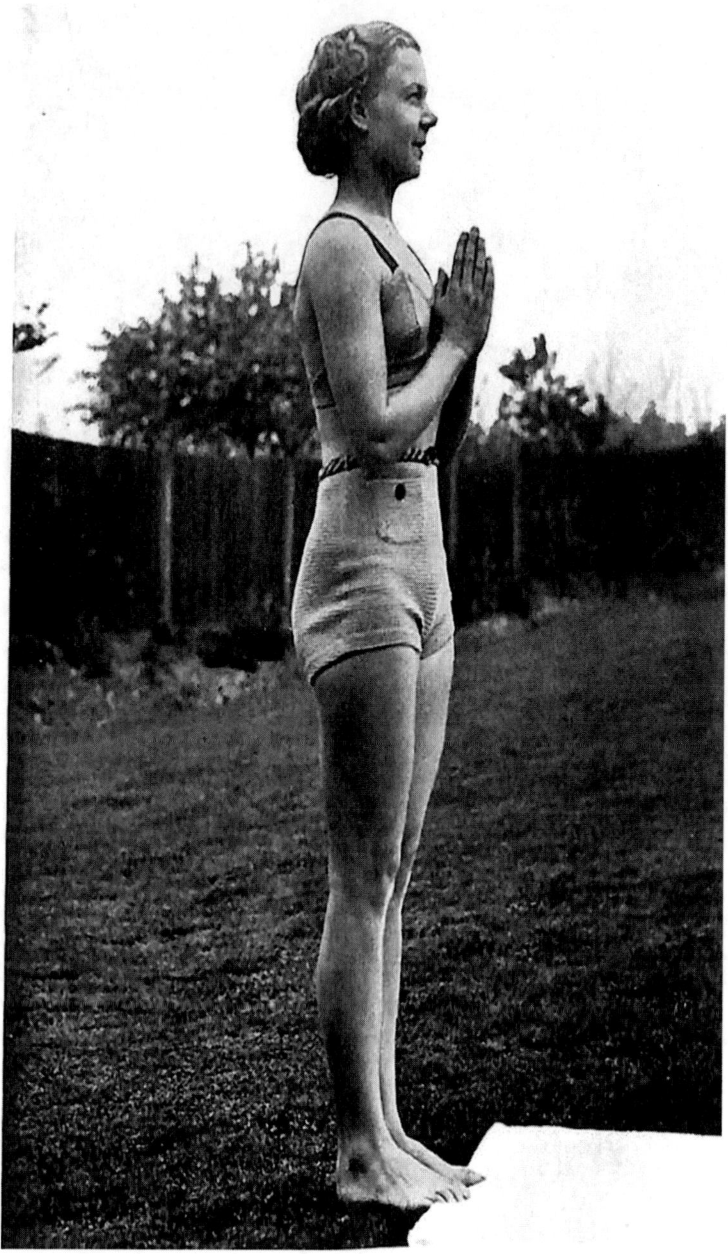

1 The starting position. Miss Brynteson has not done Surya Namaskars for long, and is not yet perfect.

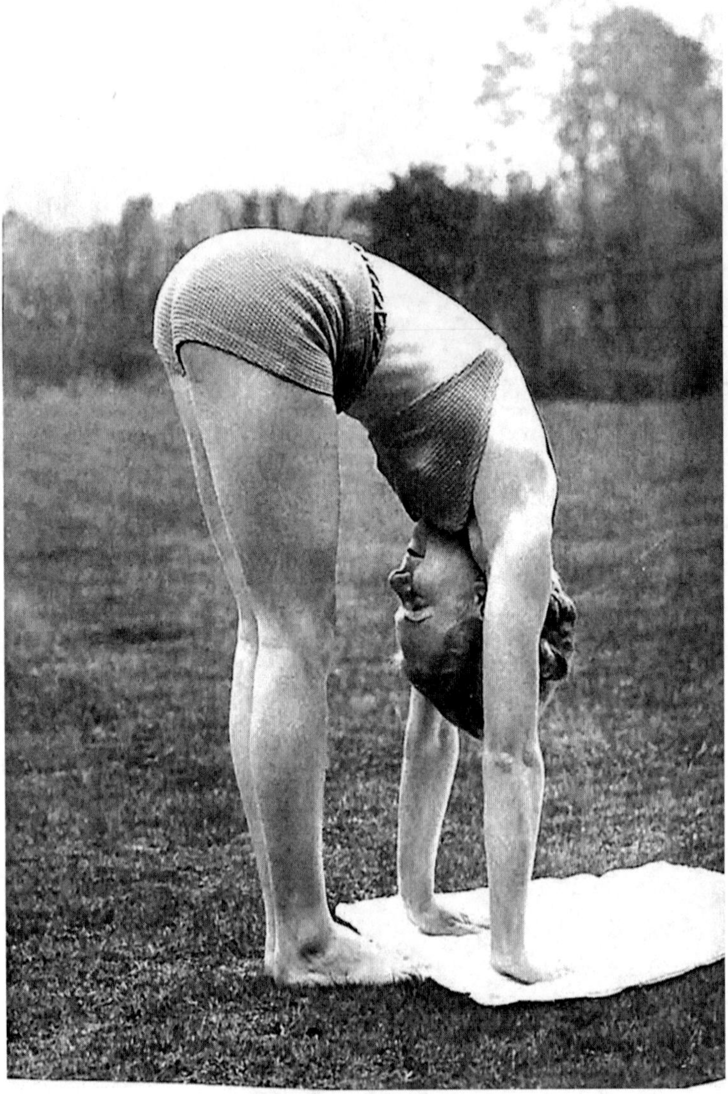

2 Hands too far away from feet. Head not touching knees. Compare this position with Appasahib's.

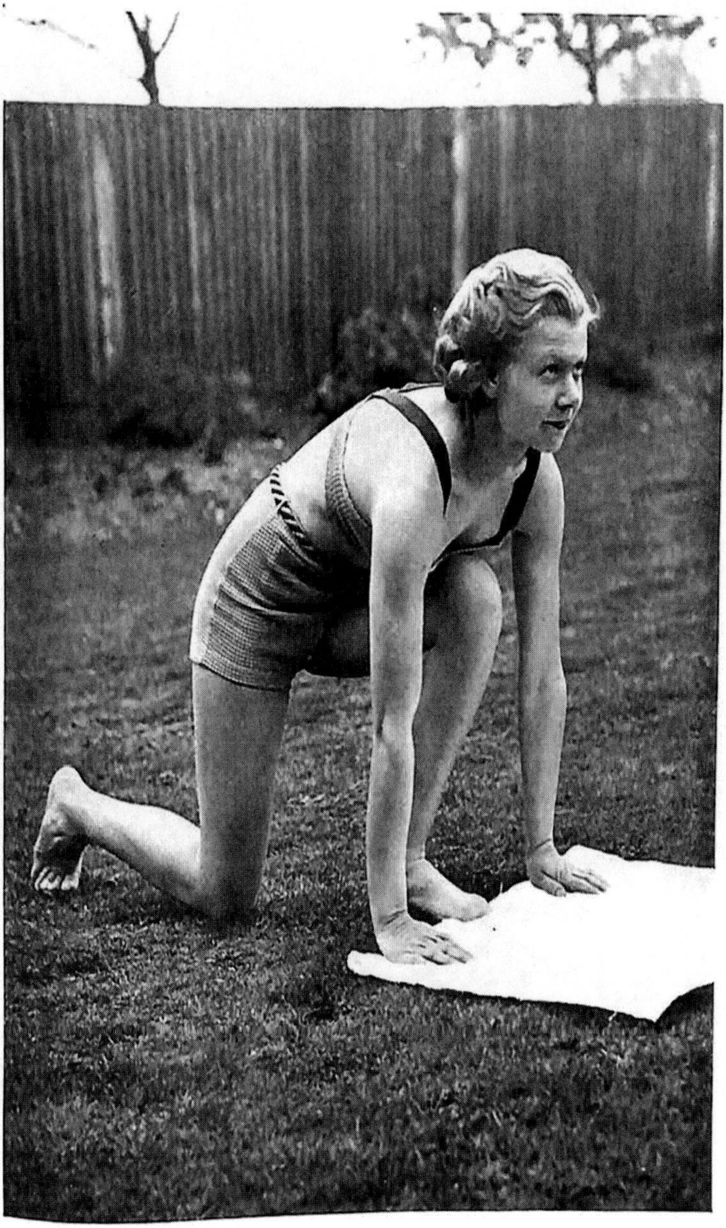

3 Perfect demonstration. Exertion confined to thrust back of head, and firm pressure of thigh against trunk.

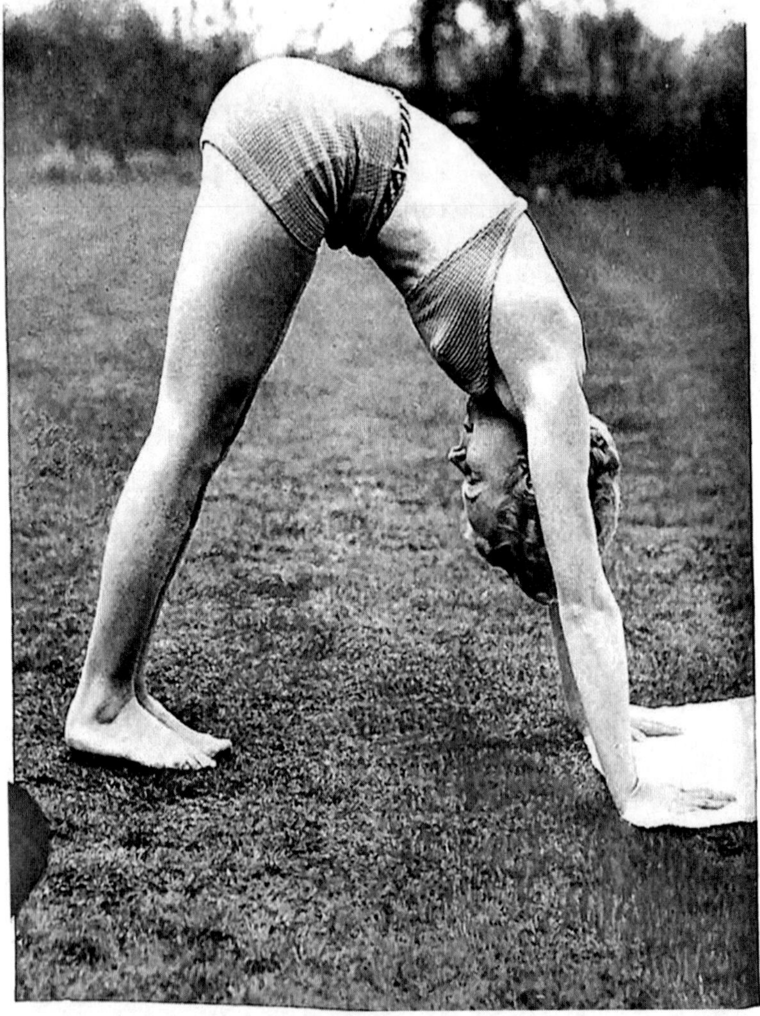

4 Back is not straight. Downward pressure at waist by helper is advisable. Net essential to keep hair in order.

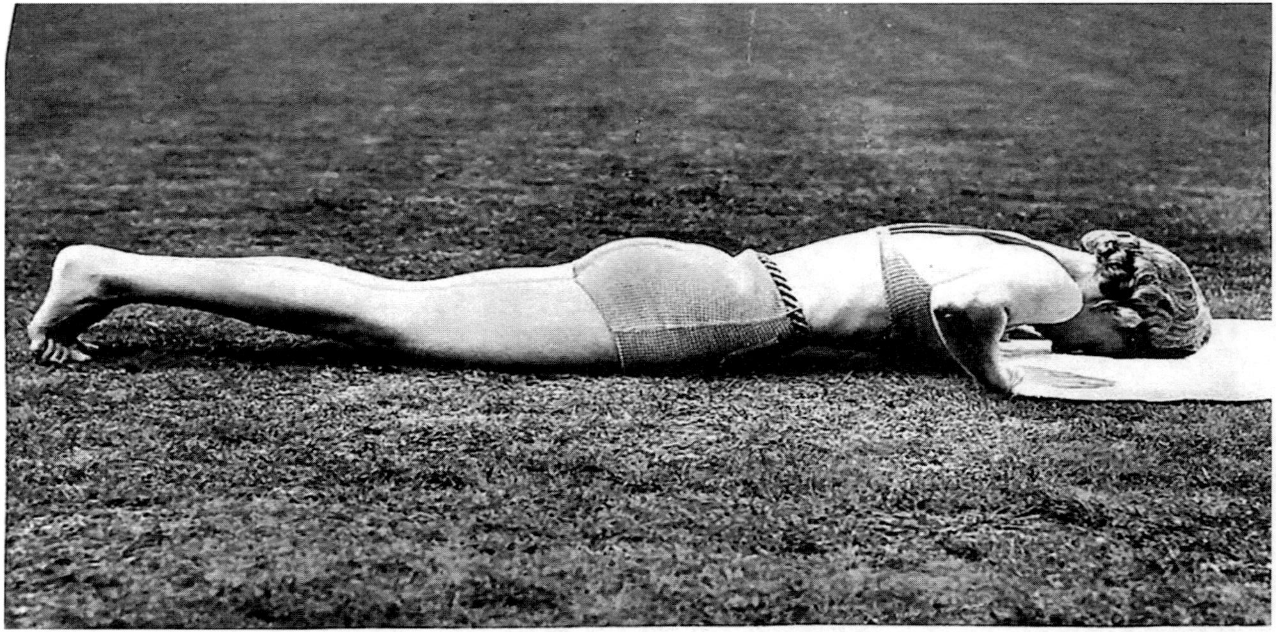

5 Note how abdomen is drawn up off ground. Toes thrust into grass. 'Looks easy, but reaches every muscle,' she said.

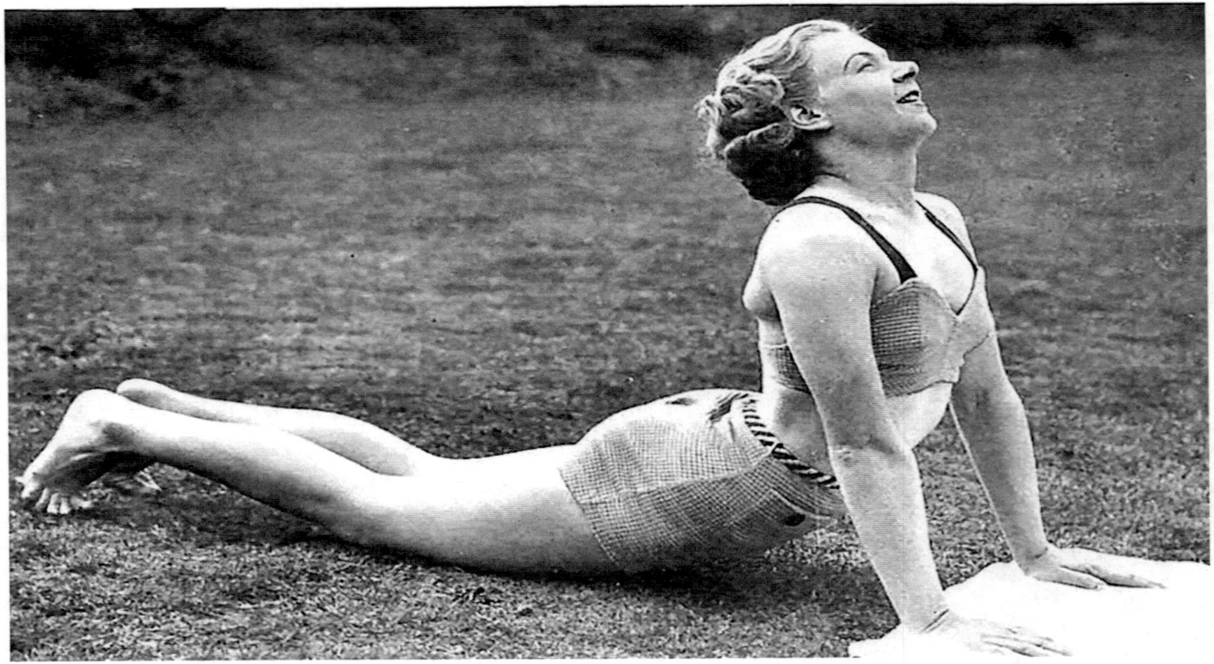

6 Sun glare made her shut her eyes. But she prefers to do the exercises out of doors in the sunlight whenever possible.

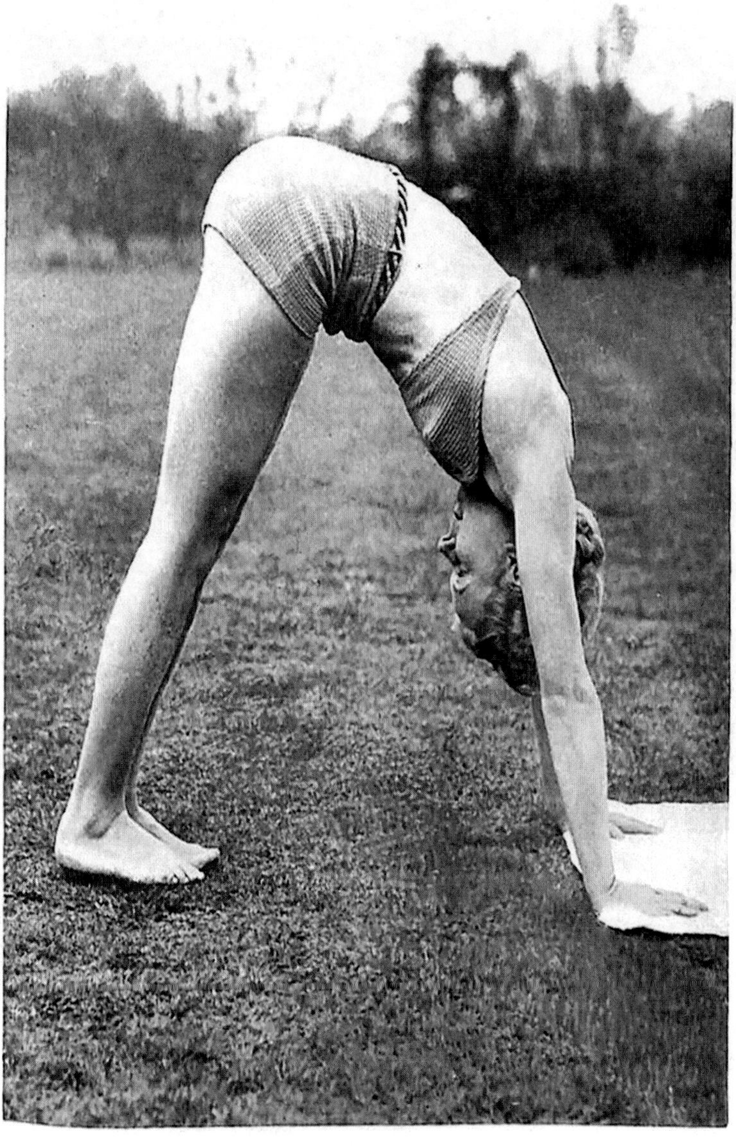

7 A wider angle between hands and feet would help attain straight line between base of spine and hands.

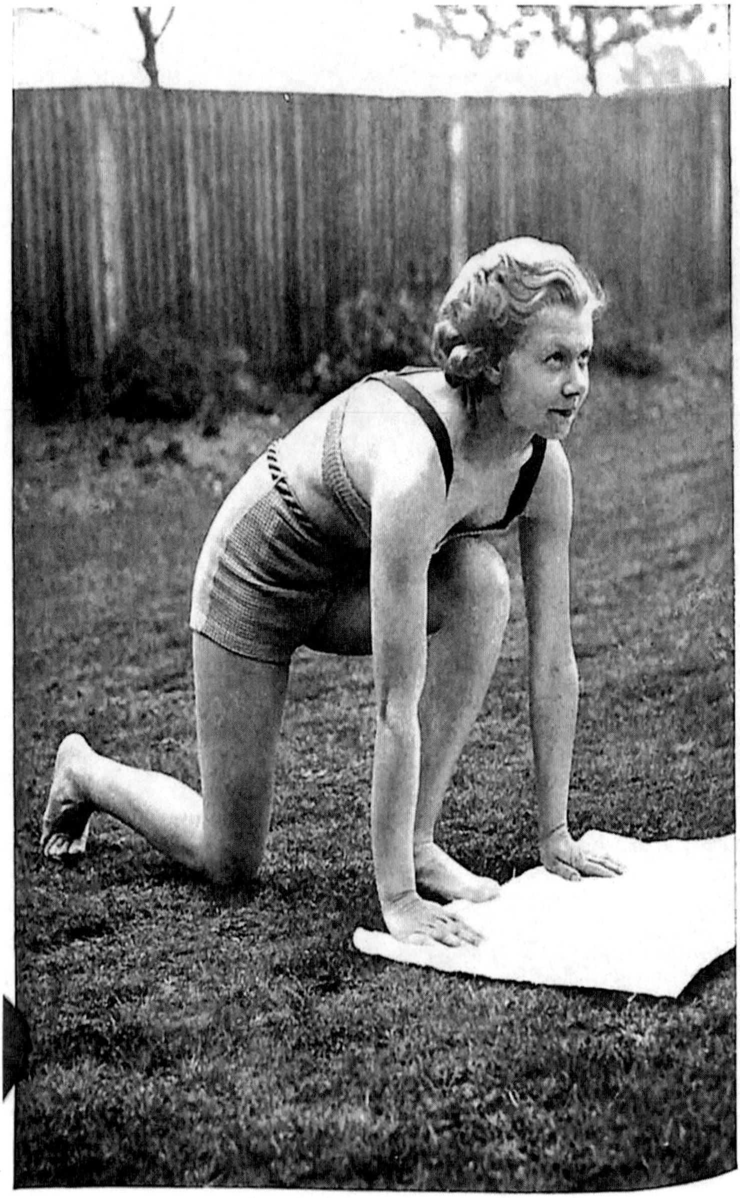

8 By this time, even on a cold day, she was warm, and intends to keep to this costume of wool and silk.

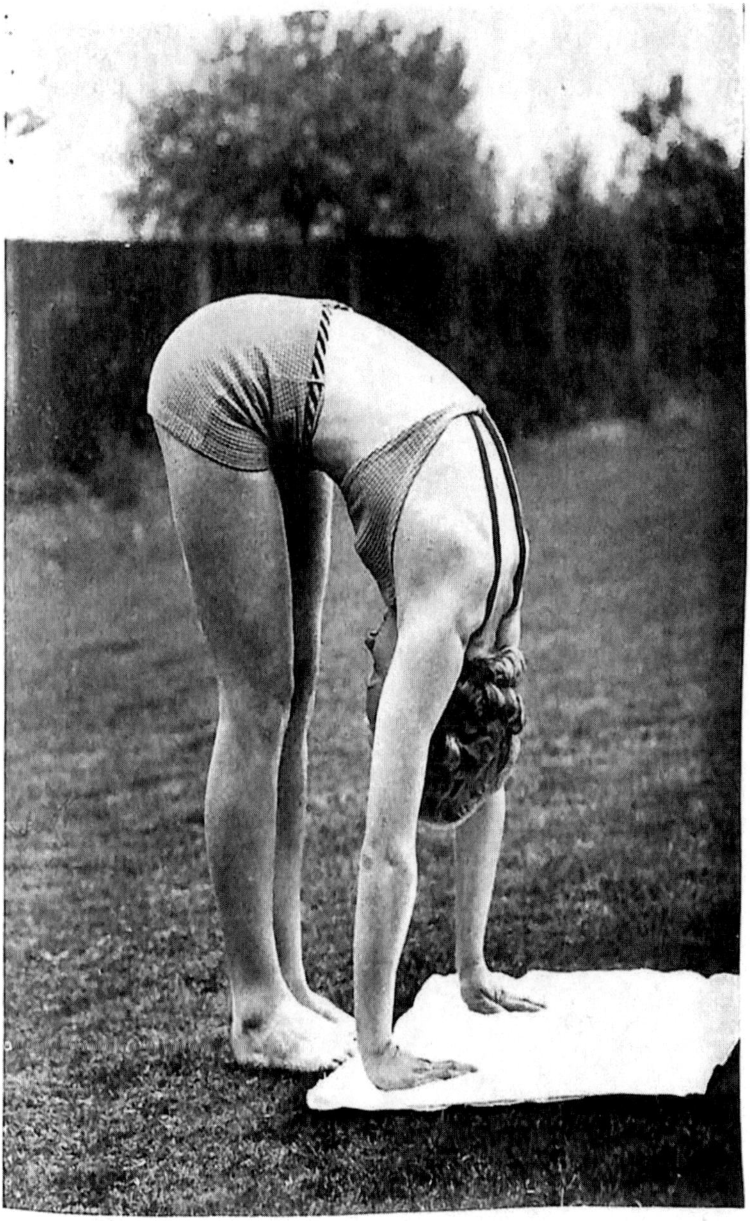

9 She has risen to this position better than she dropped to it. Next, the upward swing and deep breath.

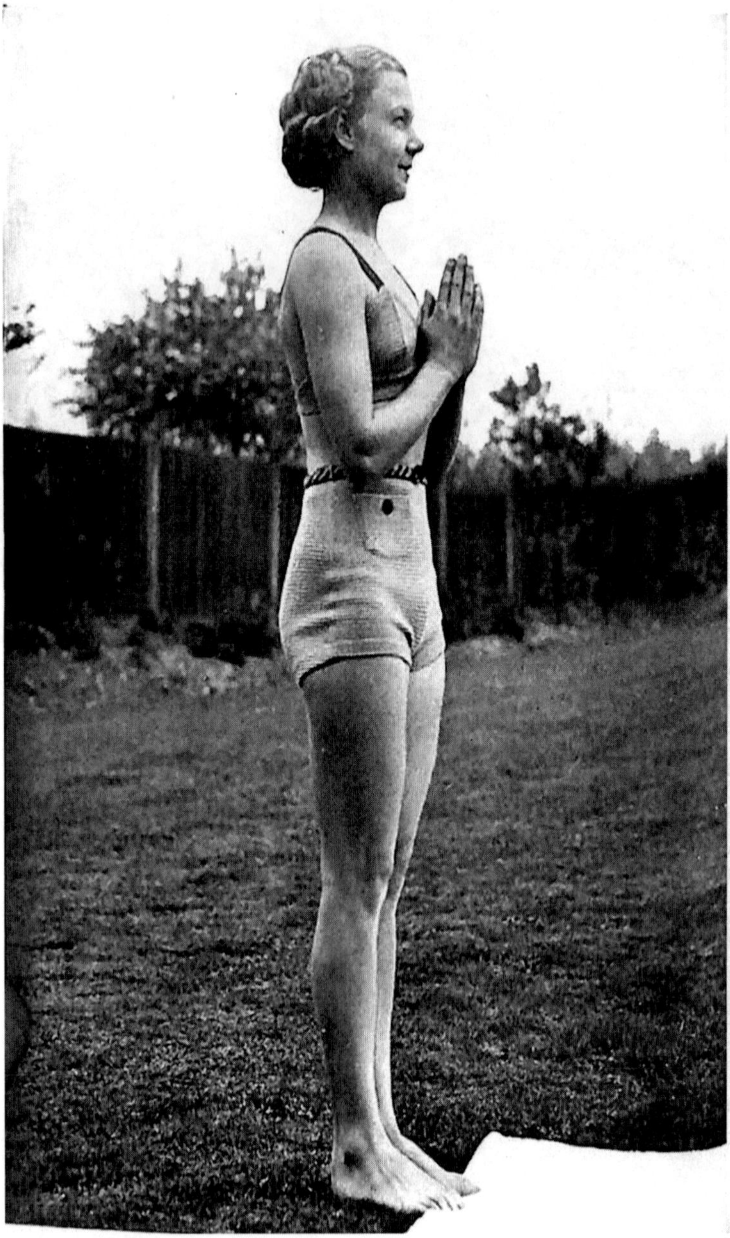

10 She will go straight on doing twenty Namaskars in five minutes—a good start for the day.

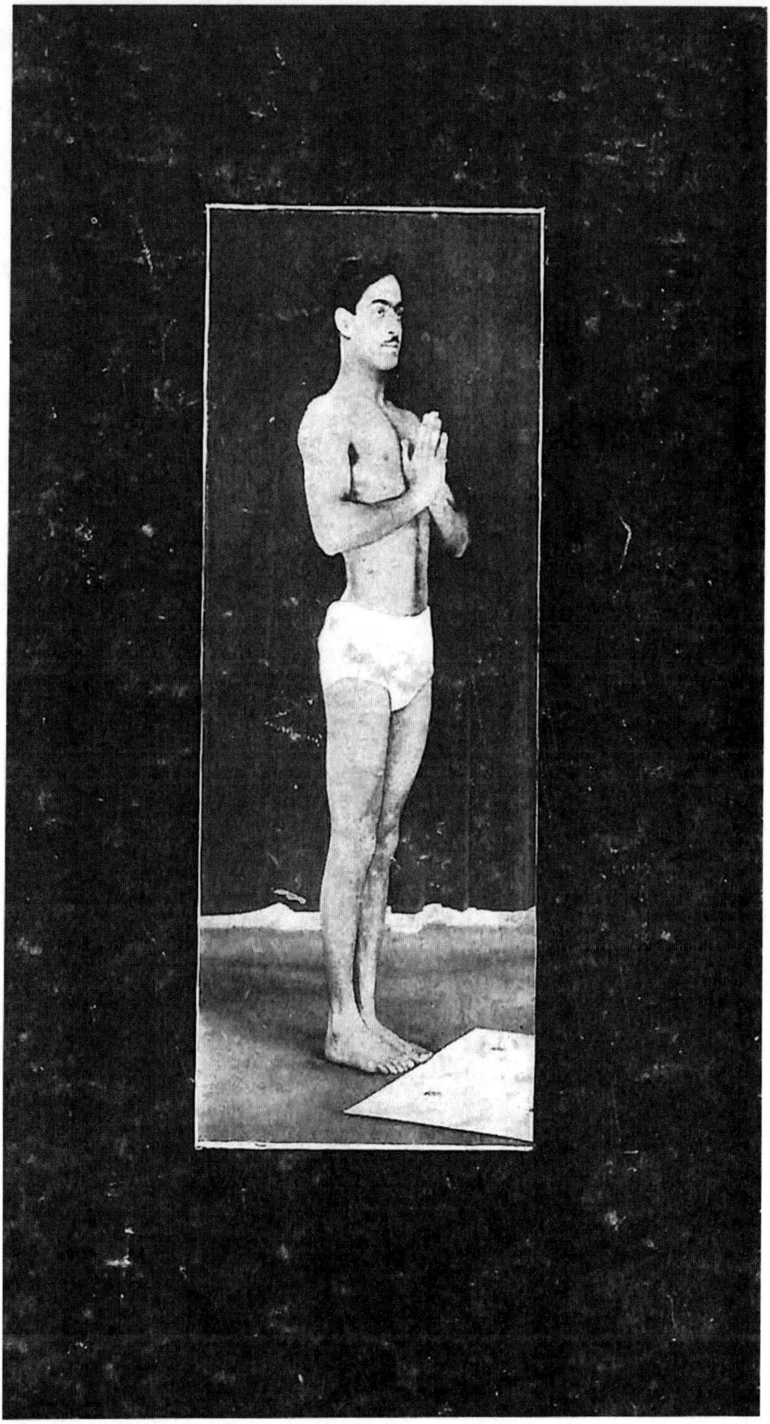